What others have said about
THE HELP PROGRAM

In order for doctors to be effective they need to HELP themselves. I use all the components of this program myself and strongly recommend them to my patients. Each segment of HELP contributes toward the process of regaining and maintaining health.

Dr Daniel Lewis, former President of the Australian Arthritis Foundation

"The HELP approach is a valuable one whether you are suffering from a specific ailment or taking preventative steps to insure your overall health and well-being. The integrated approach and practical techniques have been of great help to me."

Dr Steven Sommer, President of the Whole Health Institute

An interesting and informative book which covers a wide variety of lifestyle issues. It will be of great benefit to anyone seeking help in reducing the stresses of daily living.

Dr Vivienne Elton, psychiatrist

Our health carries messages from the depth of our psyche. In not listening to them, a state of imbalance is created. I have found that HELP creates a valuable space to listen and cater for these unrecognized needs.

Veronique Boulangier, psychologist and psychotherapist

I have never been happier than I am today thanks to the techniques I learned from this book. Less stress, and my energy level is better than ever. I feel great due to spending time each day using the HELP components. It's easy and certainly makes my life more enjoyable. I have encouraged literally thousands of people to discover the benefits of HELP through my presentations.

***Daniel Johnson, co-author of* How to Motivate, Manage and Market Yourself**

ABOUT

THE AUTHORS

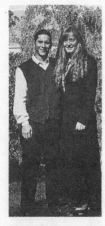

Neal Hoptman is Program Director and Health Enhancement Facilitator at the Ontos Health Retreat in East Gippsland, Victoria, Australia. He has been running programs in health enhancement for over a decade for a wide range of audiences. Previously a lecturer and researcher in the United States, he became involved in the area of holistic health and Integral Yoga, and is now sharing his training and experience through daily programs at Ontos. He is a health enhancement lifestyle consultant at hospitals, and runs seminars and workshops in Melbourne, Sydney and overseas. He has worked with the Whole Health Institute, and the Anti-Cancer Council through the auspices of the Victorian Health Promotions Foundation. Neal Hoptman along with others has now established the HELP Foundation, Inc., a non-profit charitable organization to provide education and programs to schools and the community, to complement the Health Enhancement Lifestyle Program being run in hospitals, Ontos, and businesses.

Carla Hoptman is a Health Enhancement Facilitator at the Ontos Health Retreat with a specialty in food awareness issues, healing therapies, and Integral Yoga. For many years Carla was the coordinator of the famous Ontos cuisine, and author of the popular book *Vegetarian Cookery—A Redhead in the Kitchen*. Her delicious recipes and fun approach to cooking have made for popular workshops. She is currently involved in running the Healing Arts Centre at Ontos using a wide variety of techniques to promote physical ease and mental peace. Carla also teaches yoga and meditation, both in the peaceful setting of Ontos where she lives and through workshops in the city.

HELP

YOURSELF TO HEALTH

HELP

YOURSELF TO HEALTH

—

The Health Enhancement
Lifestyle Program

NEAL AND CARLA HOPTMAN

MILLENNIUM
BOOKS

First published in 1996 by
Millennium Books
an imprint of E. J. Dwyer (Australia) Pty Ltd
Unit 13, Perry Park
33 Maddox Street
Alexandria NSW 2015
Australia
Phone: (02) 550 2355
Fax: (02) 519 3218

National Library of Australia
Cataloguing-in-Publication data
Hoptman, Neal, 1956-.
H.E.L.P. yourself to health: the unique health enhancement
lifestyle program for complete well-being in mind and body.

Bibliography.
ISBN 1 86429 058 7.

1. Self-care, Health. 2. Holistic medicine. I. Hoptman, Carla, 1960-.

613

Cover design by Mango Design Group
Text design by Bybowra Design Group Pty Ltd
Typset in Times 11pt by Bybowra Design Group Pty Ltd
Printed in Australia by Griffin Paperbacks, Netley, S.A.

10 9 8 7 6 5 4 3 2 1
00 99 98 97 96

A NOTE FROM
THE AUTHORS

—

The Health Enhancement Lifestyle Program (HELP) is designed to complement, not replace, any existing health treatments you may be receiving from your doctor or health professional. If you have a debilitating health condition, please notify your health-care provider before beginning this program.

HELP is available for everyone, although it is clear that people's needs are varied. Read this book as a way to expand your awareness of possible areas in your life that can be modified to improve your overall well-being. Discuss this book with your health professional to facilitate greater communication between you, and identify any areas of concern.

This book is dedicated to all our teachers,

including our parents, family, friends,

and the thousands of people we have learned

from in our retreats and classes.

—

ACKNOWLEDGMENTS

—

*H*ELP *Yourself to Health* has been the creation of literally hundreds of people with information that spans thousands of years. HELP is a result of a fortunate life in which we have been blessed with incredible opportunities for travel, personal development, and service, and daily teachings from family, friends, and acquaintances. During the course of writing we became aware of the countless people who have contributed in such diverse ways. Should this book come into the hands of anyone we have met, know that in some way this book is yours, for you have contributed to our lives and therefore this book. We thank all of you for assisting in this endless journey of growth, and hope that this book may help you along your path.

We would like to single out a few people for special thanks who will always continue to be an inspiration: our parents, David Hoptman and Molly Kaplansky, and Rosa and Robert Pizzini, who have encouraged us to follow our happiness and thirst for experience; Eileen, Fred, Katrina, Elena, Otto, Ron, Hilary and their families who have contributed far beyond their own awareness; and our grandparents and extended family who provided us with a rich childhood, which established the foundation for this book, and continue to guide us.

Thanks also to Neal's academic mentor at the Brookings Institute, Professor Doak Barnett, who explained one fateful afternoon that career changes were not irrevocable. He then shared, through his own life story, the importance of enjoying the journey and having faith about the destination.

The following people have all contributed to the development of HELP or read parts of this book and provided useful comments. Sincere thanks to Dr Danny Lewis, Doug Van Epps, Nicholas Brash,

Robert Bell, Joan Evans, Dr Sidney Bloch, Dr Patch Adams, Sue Bebarfald, Dr Steven Somer, Stephen Fiaylko, Daniel Johnson, Sandra McComb, Paul Littman, Dr Robert Gingold, James Mulcahey, Bhav Chaitanya, Veronique Boulangier, Mark Spatz, Mitra Somerville, Dr Geoffrey Rothchild, Dr Meyer Brott, Nischala Devi, Dr Sandra Hallam, Les Einhorn, Mas Rogers, Glenn Ceresoli, Margaret Trott, Dr Matthew Phillips, Michael Clough, Jaganath Carrera, Dr Lenny Thatch, Dan Hollander, Bhagavan Buritz, Lydia Marx, Jeffrey Blake, Dr Michael Nissen, Jonathan Levine, Debbie Golvan, Rodney Nissen, publisher Carol Floyd and the Millennium Books staff.

A special thanks to Fred Koch, a friend and brother, who has provided us with the opportunity to serve and help others through his vision and cocreation of Ontos, a unique place in which to live and work.

We have a great debt to all the Ontos Health Retreat guests who have come to our classes and HELP programs over the years, and encouraged us with their enthusiasm and progress in health enhancement. To Claire-lise and the boys without whom Ontos and this book wouldn't be the same. Thanks to Tony Jacobs, Mark Jarvis, Johnny Didge Matthews, Ian Raymond, and all the wonderful helpers, staff, and WWOOFers at Ontos over the years, who have shared their ideas and enthusiasm, and helped to keep Ontos growing while we have been developing HELP.

The practical application of Eastern thought through the yoga tradition has been a major catalyst in our lives and for this project. We would like to express our deepest gratitude to Sri Swami Satchidananda, who has been our teacher and friend over the past 12 years, for his inspiration and sharing of the precepts of Integral Yoga, which forms the basis for much of what is expressed here. The influence of these teachings in our lives is beyond words.

FIGURES

—

CONTENTS

—

reflection • Activating mind/body harmony • The humor
prescription • Weekly schedule

FOREWORD

———

BY JULIE STAFFORD

When my first book, *A Taste of Life,* was published in 1983, there were very few alternative health books available. The traditional approach to health involved standard diets, conventional exercise, and the attitude that health was something that doctors would fix up when things went awry. The explosion of interest that met my book taught me an important lesson—that people were hungry for natural good health. In the years since then, we've come a long way. The idea that 'prevention is better than a cure' has taken firm hold, and men and women today willingly participate in and take more responsibility for their own well-being.

The HELP program represents another milestone in our path toward knowledge and self-reliance in health matters. I loved reading *HELP Yourself to Health* because it is an 'action' book, not just another 'feel-good' book. Without action there is no progress, and Neal and Carla Hoptman have provided a gentle, easy method to rediscover health that speaks to everyone. Reading their book is like attending a workshop, but with one important difference—you 'attend' within your own environment and you work at your own pace.

Many of us have problems evaluating our own health, and deciding what are the most appropriate and achievable changes we can make. We've been through the vigorous aerobic stage, we've tried the fad diets, we've made and broken a thousand resolutions about healthy living. It is now half time at the ball game, and what's the score? *HELP Yourself to Health* shows you how to find out what the score is, and, by making small but significant changes to different areas of your life, to put the score in your favor—for the rest of your life.

Everyone should learn the skills that are taught in this book—in fact, they are basic health survival skills that we should be taught at school. Learning how to relax; how to eat well for well-being; how to exercise in a gentle, sustainable fashion; how to create and maintain a beautiful and calming environment... these are all important and life-enhancing skills that work together to create a balance of good health and well-being.

This holistic approach is vital, because it is only by making changes that are integral to our whole lives that we achieve the results we want. So if you've been discouraged or disheartened about achieving better health, I encourage you to try the HELP program. It shines out a message of self-reliance but shows you just how easy it can be, taking you on a step-by-step journey toward happiness and vibrant health.

Julie Stafford

PREFACE

—

W hen I completed my training as a rheumatologist specializing in problems and diseases of the musculo-skeletal system I spent most of my time dealing with the issues of diagnosis and medical treatment. Every day I would come up against seemingly insurmountable difficulties where the treatment tools at my disposal were unable to influence the suffering of my patients. Their pain was nearly always associated with distress and soon I too was becoming distressed and stressed by the limitations of my work. I realized my education needed to be broadened beyond my traditional training. This led me to search for and to discover a variety of different approaches, most of which in one way or another were connected with the holistic wisdom of past generations and different cultures.

During this time I met Neal and Carla Hoptman at the Ontos Health Retreat. It was there in the foothills of the Snowy Mountains that I was introduced by them to the Health Enhancement Lifestyle Program. This program in so many ways aligns itself with the World Health Organization's mandate for health which suggests that health includes a person's social, psychological, emotional and spiritual well-being.

Over the past eight years I have worked with Neal and Carla who have helped me to deepen my understanding and appreciation of the techniques and value of the practices of stress release, meditation, food awareness, mind/body harmony, breathing techniques, yoga, support groups, communication, time management, and the other HELP components. Practicing each of the components and integrating them as a whole has been a wonderful experience which has taught me how to look after myself—and how to be more open, available and useful to my patients.

The use of these tools has led to such positive outcomes both for myself and my patients that I have now helped establish a Department of Complementary Therapy at the Cedar Court Rehabilitation Hospital in Melbourne. Within this department HELP is offered as an integrated and complete program and is the central focus of the department. With the assistance of the Hoptmans, we are integrating all of the 12 HELP components together with the traditional and essential medical therapies available at the hospital.

At the time of this writing the introduction of HELP into the hospital has become a reality. The staff and patients at Cedar Court are now being educated in each of the 12 components of HELP included in this book. Even Australian health insurance companies are considering covering HELP for their clients.

It is an exciting development and a first in Australia, that a hospital has gone holistic in its approach. This is certainly a sign of things to come. Here in Australia and around the world medical schools are now teaching the HELP concepts that I discovered only after completing my formal medical education. I have no doubt that the pace of change will quicken. Hospital administrators here in Australia have been watching the international trends in health care over the last ten years and see that HELP is a comprehensive complementary therapy that brings together the best of ancient wisdom and modern medical research in a way that *empowers* the individual to participate in their own healing process.

Empowerment of the individual is the key if lifestyle change is to be effective. Gone are the days when patients can expect to be "cured" by their doctor without taking into account both the positive and negative effects of their daily routines, lifestyle, thought processes and emotional states. The beauty of HELP is its no-nonsense approach to the learning of effective techniques that everyone can implement over time.

This program is not only being implemented in health retreats and hospitals but at the time of this writing even school systems have expressed interest in using HELP as a vehicle for teaching health education to children.

This program emphasizes so importantly the need to begin slowly and to take small incremental steps—to give people who are unfamiliar with complementary health care time to become more familiar with a holistic approach to wellness. It is also important that individuals embark on such a program in consultation with their health practitioner as this program is not an alternative to traditional care.

This book is a very useful guide. In providing both the detailed steps to health enhancement as well as practical suggestions for daily life, everyone can begin to usher in a more easeful body, a peaceful mind, and a useful life. Both myself and my family and those of my patients who have already been trained by Neal and Carla in HELP attest to the effectiveness of this approach.

A health-enhancing lifestyle program is the best medical insurance a person can have. By taking responsibility for our own health and by using the experience and skills of medical practitioners in a complementary manner, we get the ideal environment not only for disease management but for disease prevention and improvement in quality of life.

I recommend HELP to my patients and my colleagues, after having experienced the benefits myself. It is my firm belief that we are not just helping ourselves to health. When we look after our own health we are also giving a gift to our families, our community, and the world around us.

Dr Daniel Lewis MBBS FRACP
Former President of
The Australian Arthritis Foundation

INTRODUCTION

—

ABOUT THIS BOOK — AND HOW TO USE IT

The HELP approach is accessible to all: people who find themselves in a crisis scenario, and those who want to have a healthier and more integrated lifestyle. The program is both preventive and an effective means of rehabilitation for those seeking to remedy damage already done. HELP also assists in decreasing the likelihood of future occurrences of disease by altering the underlying factors that may contribute to health challenges.

The fundamental concept is one of balancing our lives through the integration of a number of easy-to-implement practical steps, which will enable us to avoid the pitfalls of both environmental pressures and genetic weaknesses—pressures that we fall prey to when we lack balance in our lives. While many approaches to health focus on a particular technique of health care, such as aerobic exercise or stress reduction, the approach taken in this book is integrative and holistic. No one particular component is sufficient to bring balance unless all other factors in our lives are already in harmony. Despite good intentions, just changing what we eat, for example, will not of itself reverse dis-ease unless the other factors that account for the problem are addressed as well.

By adopting HELP we can still maintain our responsibilities and commitments, but at the same time bring these into balance with our health requirements. While we are often seduced by the simplicity of adding just one new technique to our daily lives and hoping that it will be a panacea for the variety of ills or potential ills facing us, it is unrealistic to think that a single technique will work at a fundamental level. The approach taken here requires us to have an awareness and acceptance of where we find ourselves at this present moment, and then, through an understanding of the diverse underlying factors that account for this present position, to make a commitment to adjust our lives to usher in well-being.

HOW TO HELP YOURSELF

Each chapter of this guide contains one of the elements of the HELP format, providing an introduction to the subject, as well as practical instructions and guidance on how to incorporate it into your daily life. Before making a commitment to the program it is essential to understand each of the components fully, to reflect honestly on your current lifestyle approach, and then to develop an action strategy to integrate the program into your daily life. Understanding, reflection, and action are thus the three key mental directives when reading each chapter.

Understanding

Given the entrenched nature of our current lifestyle patterns, it is vital to fully understand each component of the program before making any changes. It must make sense to you in relation to your present life. You should feel confident in explaining each component to other people who might challenge, question, or be interested in finding out more regarding the changes you are making in your life. HELP is an action-oriented program. While there is not a great emphasis on the theory behind each component, there is a tremendous amount of research that has been done on each aspect of the program. If you would like to pursue this information further, please make use of the Further Reading section at the end of each chapter.

This is not a program to be taken on faith, and that is why understanding HELP is so important. Only through being aware of the validity of each component, and seeing how the components complement one another, will it be possible to make a commitment to the program and derive full benefit from it. This is a dynamic and interactive program, which will bring greater benefits to you as your understanding of and commitment to each element of the program deepen.

Reflection

Once you fully understand the particular component described in each chapter, take time to reflect on your current daily lifestyle and the degree to which this aspect of the program is a vital part of your life.

This is a very important stage, as it is an indicator of your starting point for the program and of where change needs to take place. Some of you may already be incorporating some elements of the program in your daily life to varying degrees, and may need to make fewer changes than others. A period of honest reflection will enable you to evaluate the specific changes that can be made to derive full benefit from that component.

A HELP Journal

When going through the reflection section of each chapter, you will find it useful to establish a HELP journal in which you can write down your reflections. The journal will be a record to allow you to monitor your progress, record your current state of health, allow you to express feelings that arise, and uplift your spirits.

A loose-leaf folder with lined paper and 12 dividers is all you need to start. Photocopy the pages in Appendix 2 and place each one behind the appropriate divider of the components of HELP:

- Releasing Stress
- Physical Exercise
- An Easeful Body
- A Quality Environment
- Food Awareness
- Mind/Body Connection
- Breath of Life
- A Peaceful Mind
- Creative Expression and Learning
- Group Support and Communication

- Service

- Planning Health Enhancement

When recording your reflections, begin each entry with the date, time of day, your location, and any specific thoughts regarding your physical, mental, emotional, and spiritual well-being on that day. You will find this information helpful when examining your journal over a period of time. Feel free to be creative and incorporate drawings, memories, objects from nature, or anything else that comes to mind. A personal HELP journal is a catalyst for the creative process and it can take many forms. Let your imagination run free. Use the journal to keep track of your personal health goals, and refine and evaluate them over time.

Once you have been involved in the program for some time, it is often easy to lose track of the dramatic changes that have taken place as you fine-tune your lifestyle; the changes become more subtle. When glancing back through your journal after some time you will be reminded of your base point, and it will be a motivating tool to keep you on track. Do not underestimate the importance of reflection and recording your insights in the journal—it is an essential part of your progress and an investment in the future.

Action

The final step is the development of an action-oriented strategy for implementing the program. Each chapter includes detailed instructions on how to incorporate that component into your daily life, with practical steps and HELPful hints that are easy to implement given dedication and commitment. Putting the program into action will naturally follow from an understanding of each element, reflection on where you are starting from, and the setting of realistic goals.

Remember the SAME rule when setting goals. Each goal should be:

- Specific

- Achievable

- Measurable

- Enjoyable

There is no quicker way to lose momentum than to set up a rigorous program that requires a complete upheaval in your daily schedule and is too ambitious to achieve in your current circumstances. This will leave you with a sense of disappointment and failure. Remember, it is better to achieve 75 percent of your potential regularly than 100 percent inconsistently. In addition to the suggestions at the conclusion of each chapter, the planning section at the end of the book will assist you in developing a schedule that works for you.

In each section of your journal, set up an achievable daily "to do" list that includes a practical step from each chapter (e.g. "I will do 25 minutes of walking daily"). If for some reason you do not have the opportunity to implement all of the items on the list, do not chastise yourself incessantly. Rather, see to it that this commitment is carried forward to the following day to gain both the benefit as well as a sense of completion. It may take some time before you can incorporate all components in your life. Achieving small quality steps is the key to a successful long-term program.

As available time and your ability allow the "to do" list to grow, occasionally expand your goals. Remember to be realistic, writing down any changes required for these new goals. This approach will ensure steady progress with a cumulative impact on your overall quality of life that will be lasting in its transformational effects. To maintain motivation and share the benefits you may wish to set goals with family members and friends, or join a local group.

The degree to which you apply these principles of understanding, reflection, and action will determine your success in developing a health-enhancing lifestyle. This is not a competition, and your action strategy should not leave you feeling as if you are in an endurance test. Even if the changes are small and slow to begin with, remember that they are headed in a positive direction. Enjoy the journey. Challenge yourself, but do not strain or put yourself under such pressure that the program loses its sense of fun and adventure.

Releasing STRESS

—

UNDERSTANDING STRESS

When exploring the subject of stress and how to reduce, release, and manage it, it is essential to take some time to understand a little about stress. First, we must understand that stress is not something outside of ourselves. Stress is our reaction to change. That is why two people can go through exactly the same event but have completely different responses. This is a very important point, because if stress is our reaction to an event, we can work on changing it; whereas if stress were a random event outside of ourselves, we would be at its mercy.

For example, though work may become easier through technological innovation, stress is not necessarily eliminated. Stress is an internal response to external change, and such change is a fact of life and therefore can not be eliminated regardless of the modernization of society. Some might also argue that the accelerating rate of technological change in recent years has triggered greater stressful reactions. Such generalizations are difficult to prove, but by developing a greater awareness of stress as our own reaction to change, we can develop techniques to help us alter our perception of stressful factors outside of ourselves in an ever-changing world.

But not all stress is bad or harmful. Stress can be a significant motivating force in our daily lives. It is only when we begin to pass over that fine line that divides motivation from frustration that the techniques for releasing stress become important for overall health and well-being. Awareness of the role of stress in our daily lives, both as a tool and as a debilitating force, is the key. If we can reduce the destructive stress responses, then our overall health will be greatly benefited.

REFLECTING ON STRESS

A great deal of our blockage with stressful situations is a direct result of our perspective. If we could step outside of the immediate situation and view it as an outsider, we could begin to reduce this stress. To what degree does your perception of limited time contribute to your stress response? Take a moment to reflect back and visualize a time when you felt stressed. Maybe you had an important appointment, and you were running late through no fault of your own. Then you found yourself locked in traffic with the clock ticking away. Your teeth clenched, your heart beat faster, maybe you were muttering to yourself, and your breathing was rapid and shallow. Yet a week later it was an event that you could hardly remember. This physiological reaction to the perception of stress is part of what is known as the fight-or-flight response of the body. But this response is not involuntary; we can alter it through our mental perspective on changes in our environment.

Through being aware of the role that time plays in producing a stress response as well as giving us perspective on situations in the past, we can begin the process of acceptance. To be able to say, yes, I am running late for my appointment. Yes, I am unfortunately caught up in an awful traffic jam. And yes, this appointment is very important. However, I must accept that all these factors are beyond my control at the moment and in a week I will hardly remember this event, so let me witness the situation from that perspective now, and do my best with what is in my control rather than compounding it by my reaction. In addition to the psychological relief gained from this approach, the physiological effect can be dramatic as the body remains relaxed with no gnashing of teeth, no increase in blood pressure, no constriction of the chest and speeding up of the heartbeat, and no release of stress hormones such as cortisol.

Take a moment to recall a recent stress response that you have had. Clearly go through the details of the situation that you found yourself in and record them in your journal. How did the stress response manifest itself in your body? Make a list in your journal of the sensations you felt, such as rapid heartbeat, shallow and fast breathing, and any feelings you experienced, such as anger, resentment, frustration, helplessness. Now reflect on how the situation was resolved and recall the lessons that you learned.

Develop the habit of reflecting back on stressful moments in your life and recording your reaction in your journal. As you practice the

techniques outlined in this chapter notice how your reactions change.
Keep the format of your journal entries the same so that you can
easily compare your stress response over time.

The following format may be useful:

• Details of the stress-response situation

• Physical reaction

• Feelings experienced

• Resolution

• Lessons

Once we are outside the immediate situation that provoked the stress
response, it seems far easier to be philosophical about the event, and
oftentimes to see the positive results that came about because of it.
The trick is to gain this perspective in the moment, and that requires
us to develop the capacity to witness the body and the mind, and then
to experience the peaceful nature within us that is often clouded by
our reactions. Progressive deep relaxation is a technique that performs
this educational role of giving us experience of the witness state, as
well as allowing us to release tension and stress from the body and
mind through coming in touch with our peaceful essence. As with the
other components of HELP, the key is to practice it regularly.

PROGRESSIVE DEEP RELAXATION

The progressive deep relaxation technique is one of the physical
practices of hatha yoga. It allows the body to heal and repair itself. It
helps us to release stress, reduce anxiety, and remove mental blocks.
It has a variety of applications in the area of psychology, helping to
relieve insomnia, assisting the mind in absorbing new learning
materials, and allowing the natural tendency of the body to heal to
come forth without impediments.

It is based on the principle that a muscle will relax more profoundly
when you tense it first. It begins with exaggerating any tension in the
body through contraction of the muscles in different parts of the body,

then relaxing both the exaggerated tension as well as any underlying tension that had been there to begin with.

The format of the progressive relaxation described here includes:

- Assuming a comfortable horizontal position
- Stretching and tightening muscles from the toes to the head
- Releasing and relaxing muscles
- Mentally scanning the entire body
- Being aware of the breathing
- Letting go of mental distractions
- Being aware of the peace within
- Slowly stretching and awakening the body

To prepare for this practice, find a quiet, comfortable location in which you will not be disturbed for at least 15 minutes. You may want to have a blanket nearby as the body temperature tends to drop as the body relaxes, and perhaps a cushion or two for comfort. Now lie down on your back. Scan the body first and adjust your clothing so that you feel completely comfortable. Feel free to place cushions either behind the head or underneath the back of the knees to release pressure on the lower back. Make whatever changes are necessary for you to feel at ease. Adjust your position so that your feet are roughly shoulder width apart. Your arms are slightly away from the body with the palms facing up. The head is in a comfortable position, and the eyes are gently closed. Start with a full deep inhalation followed by a slow relaxed exhalation.

EXERCISE

Become aware of any sounds that you can hear and just identify the sound, let it go, and move on to the next. Not getting caught up in any one sound as you bring your awareness slowly within.

Next tune into your breathing and become aware of the rhythm of the breath. The sound of the breath as it enters and leaves the body. The rise and fall of the chest. Just allow the breathing to relax fully.

Now bring the awareness to the right leg and foot, stretching them out, tensing the muscles in the leg and foot, raising them slightly up off the floor, tensing the muscles tighter, then releasing. Allow the leg to come to a comfortable position and forget all about it as you now follow the same procedure for the left leg.

Now inhale deeply and contract the muscles of your buttocks, tensing the muscles tighter, as tight as you can, then just release, allowing the buttocks to sink into the floor.

Then bring the awareness to your abdominal area. Expand the abdomen out like a balloon as you take in a full deep breath, take in a little more air, a little more air, then hold onto the breath. Open the mouth and let the air come rushing out with a whooshing sound. Now do the same with the chest as you take in a deep breath, expanding out the chest, taking in a little more air, a little more air, then holding onto the breath. Open the mouth and let the air come rushing out, feeling the chest area free up and relax completely.

Now become aware of your right arm and hand. Stretch them out, splaying out the fingers, then make a fist as you tense the muscles of the hand and the arm, raising them slightly off the floor as you tense the muscles tighter, tighter, then release, allowing the arm and hand to relax. Find a comfortable position for the arm, uncurling the fingers, and feel the right arm let go as you repeat the process for the left arm.

Leaving your arms relaxed, bring your awareness to the shoulders as you tense the muscles around the shoulders, raising them up toward the ears, then down toward the feet, then trying to bring the shoulders together toward a point at the center of the chest, then letting go and releasing the shoulders, allowing them to relax down.

Gently roll your head from side to side, and as you do so relax all the muscles of the neck. Now find a comfortable position for the head and just allow it to rest there.

Become aware of the facial muscles by opening and closing the jaw a few times. Then purse the lips, wrinkle the nose, and squint the eyes. Finally, raise the eyebrows and furrow the forehead. Then just let the facial muscles relax.

Next make any adjustments to your position, cushions, blanket, or clothing, and make a commitment to remain still, as you scan the body mentally to release any subtle tension that may still remain. Begin by visualizing the toes of both feet and sending the signal for any tension to let go as you mentally free up the toes. Then work your way through the rest of the body: soles of the feet, heels, tops of the feet, ankles, shins, calf muscles, knees, thighs, buttocks, back region, abdomen, chest, hands, arms, shoulders, neck, and facial muscles. Just visualize and relax all these parts in turn.

Now bring the awareness back to the breath. Become aware of how peaceful and relaxed the breathing has become as you attune to the breath, and just witness the breathing.

Next become aware of the mind—any thoughts, images or ideas passing through the mind. Project them onto an imaginary screen. Now just let them pass from that screen, not getting caught up in the thoughts or images. A silent witness to the mind.

Now focus on the peace within. Become aware of how peaceful the body, the breath, and the mind have become. This peace is your true nature. Merge in with this peace, become one with this peace, feel the peace, and just enjoy it.

After a few minutes begin to deepen the breathing and feel the body being energized and refreshed with each deep breath. Begin to awaken the body slowly by gently moving the toes, the fingers, the legs, stretching out the arms, rolling the head, and taking time to tune into the physical body. Once you have stretched fully, slowly come back up to a seated position.

Learning to Witness the Body

While deep relaxation is simple and straightforward, its benefits are profound. Practicing this technique leaves us feeling a sense of balance and peace. By learning to witness the body, the breath, and the mind, we cultivate the ability to bring this witness perspective into our everyday lives to reduce our stress reactions.

To witness does not mean to imply inaction or passivity. By maintaining our perspective on the big picture, we are free to be actively engaged with our environment. We are able to put whatever events or changes we are experiencing around us into a mental framework that is not constrained by the events or changes themselves. We do this all the time with things our mind considers trivial; the key is to be able to do it in situations where we harbor attachment, desires, or a sense of self-consciousness (e.g. while we might not notice or care if someone calls us by the wrong name, we might take exception to being called a derogatory name). The witness perspective will be heightened by meditative practice, as well as by other components of the HELP program.

GUIDED IMAGERY

It is possible to expand on the progressive deep relaxation by adding another component which is often referred to as imagery, or directed or creative visualization. This technique centers around the responses of the body to the images in the mind. We are all aware of this dynamic in daily life. When daydreaming of a pleasant holiday, for example, we feel the body begin to relax, the breath becoming deeper and more regular, and a sense of peace within. Or when recalling a particular conflict situation, we feel the heart speed up, the muscles tense, the breath become shallow, and the mind agitated. All these reactions are triggered just by recalling in images different scenes from life. Whether we visualize an erotic scene or imagine biting into a ripe juicy lemon, there is an accompanying physiological response, as the phenomenon of mind imagery is a powerful one.

How does this take place? The body and mind are connected by chemical messengers known as peptides. They respond to all the senses; whether the imagery involves sight, sound, touch, smell, or taste, these transmitters provide the linkage. Numerous medical studies have detailed the power of this interconnection.

The potential applications of guided imagery are unlimited. Not only are these techniques actively used in the healing field, but they have become extremely popular in sports and business, as individuals visualize upcoming challenges in as much detail as possible and then guide themselves through a successful fulfillment of those challenges. Whether it be closing a large sale, or jumping hurdles in record time at the Olympics, the success of guided imagery has led to it being actively taught in these fields as well as in many others.

Guided Imagery Techniques

You may wish to incorporate guided imagery into your progressive deep relaxation. When you have relaxed the body and are focusing on the peace is an appropriate time to introduce your imagery. The benefit of doing it at this stage is that the body, breath, and mind have been systematically relaxed and your internal awareness is heightened to respond to the images. Some people feel that introducing the imagery at this point brings them out of a relaxed state into a more actively alert frame of mind, and prefer to keep imagery separate from the relaxation. Some like to produce their own imagery, and others prefer to use a tape that will guide them through. The choice is yours, and you are encouraged to experiment with what works for you.

If you choose to use imagery outside of the deep relaxation context, then identify a time when you have a moment to just close the eyes, bring the awareness within, and let go of external distractions. While sitting or lying down in a comfortable position, just let go of sounds and sense stimuli. Scan the body to attune to it, then begin with a few deep full inhalations followed by slow relaxed and prolonged exhalations. This will allow you to let go into the imagery as much as possible.

Imagery techniques vary according to your goals, whether they be stress reduction, healing and repairing the body, improving performance, and so forth. There are several key ingredients common to all approaches which tend to enhance the success of the imagery. These should be foremost in your mind when planning imagery, as they will allow the body to respond much more effectively:

- Be clear about your goal and focus on only one goal at a time.

- Believe in your goal with full conviction.

- Feel that it is possible to realize your goal in the short term, giving it a sense of immediacy.

- Create an image of the process in full detail that will allow you to reach that goal.

- Use whatever tools will allow you to provide further detail, such as mental pictures.

- Involve all the senses—touch, taste, sound, smell, and sight—when using this imagery.

- Make a physical drawing of your goal to allow you to put in as much detail as possible.

- Now shift your goal into the present as if it already exists and you are experiencing it.

- Whenever possible, recall your goal and use that imagery to reinforce it as often as you can.

An Example of Guided Imagery

The following imagery technique is effective for letting go of stress. You could have someone read it to you, make a tape of it, or use it as a guide when conducting your own imagery exercise.

Adjust yourself so that you are sitting or lying in a comfortable position. Go through the preliminary preparation detailed on page five for bringing the awareness within, or incorporate the guided imagery exercise into your progressive deep relaxation. Your goal is to let go and release stress. You know that this is possible and can be done at this moment.

E X E R C I S E

Visualize yourself walking along the beach. Feel the sand moving with each footstep, the warmth of the sun as it caresses your skin. A gentle breeze cools and refreshes the body. Become aware of the sounds of the beach as you continue to walk along. The sound of the waves as they roll in and back out again. The sound of the seagulls as they call out to one another. Become aware of the fresh air and the accompanying scent of the sea as you breathe deeply into the lungs, as if you can taste the salt in the sea air. Become aware of all the colors around you and feel them soothe and relax your entire being. The blue of the sky. The white wisps of cloud. The blue and green of the sea. The yellow of the sun.

You are completely in the moment with each step you take along the sand. No thoughts of the past. No expectations of the future. Just being with each breath and with each step in the moment. The body feels peaceful and relaxed. The mind still and calm. You are filled with a spirit of joy as you feel at one with nature, interconnected and whole.

As you continue to walk along the beach you come to a dune and walk to the top of it, where you sit down and gaze out to sea. Despite the activity on the shoreline there is a peace and tranquillity out at sea. The waves on the beach are like the breath. Rising and falling in an endless cycle. But beyond them, deep in the sea, is a deep reservoir of peace, just like there is within you. Dive deep into this reservoir of peace and joy, and feel it completely soothe and relax the body and mind. Know that this peaceful state is your true nature. Attune to it, and come to know it. Realize that this peace is always with you no matter where you go. Take time to come in contact with it, and allow it to flow throughout your entire being.

Feel any concerns you might have being washed away with the waves, and feel renewed energy flow into the body with the rays of sunshine. Feel the body being restored and rejuvenated by nature. Attune the breath with the waves flowing in and flowing out as you become one with the rhythm. Feel the consciousness of the physical body begin to drop away, like a set of clothes falling off, leaving you with a sense of being connected with all of nature. At one with the sand, the water, the sky. Feeling whole, nourished, and sustained by the forces of nature.

As you sit atop the dune the sun slowly begins to set, sending an array of colors blazing across the sky, with orange and red reflected both in the sky and in the water below. The sun seems to disappear into the water. The bright red ball of fire descends out of view and leaves behind a magnificent masterpiece of hues. You are filled with a sense of joy at nature's beauty. You feel alive, vital, and renewed.

You make a commitment to yourself to take time out from your daily schedule to attune to this spirit of peace and joy within. To nurture it and share it with all you meet. Allowing this peace and joy to spread throughout the universe to everyone and everything.

As you descend from the dune, following your footprints in the sand, you feel a lightness throughout your entire being. You see a lone seagull soaring high above the water, framed by the beautiful colors of the sky. How effortlessly it glides on the air currents. You too feel this sense of soaring and gliding. Not being carried forth by your feet or legs, but by that spirit of peace and joy within you. Allow that spirit to stay with your awareness wherever you go and whatever is happening around you.

Begin to deepen the breath once again. Send the energy of the breath throughout the entire body as you become aware of how refreshed and peaceful the body, breath, and mind have become. Once you have attuned back to your position, slowly open your eyes.

POSITIVE AFFIRMATIONS

Another tool for transforming our lives is that of positive affirmations, or statements that we design to assist us in developing new ways of enjoying life and achieving our goals. Every thought we have carries with it a chemical reaction in the body that can influence the functioning of body and mind. A clear and positive statement regarding each of our goals can precipitate a physiological and psychological reaction, which can in turn align both the body and mind with the achievement of that goal. Medical research is now confirming the benefits of optimism, faith, and positive thinking for the body. Similar guidelines apply with regard to affirmations as to imagery:

- Be clear about your goal.

- Set only one goal at a time.

- Dedicate yourself to that goal with full commitment.

- Write the goal down in positive terms which indicate it is becoming a reality now.

- Write the goal clearly and concisely so that it can be easily repeated several times daily. This is your positive affirmation.

- Introduce your positive affirmation into your progressive deep relaxation whenever possible.

- When scheduling your daily priorities mentally or in your diary, determine whether they are conducive to your affirmation, and if not, alter them.

- Develop a sense of enthusiasm for your affirmation, bringing it into the here and now.

- Begin the day as you awake with your affirmation, and conclude each evening with it.

- If your goal changes slightly, be sure to alter the affirmation accordingly.

- Reward yourself for making the affirmation a reality in a way that is meaningful to you, before moving on to another one.

An example of a positive affirmation for stress release could be: "Each day I am able to react to changes and people around me in a more peaceful and relaxed way." Whenever you can, remind yourself of the affirmation. Write it down numerous times. Share it with others to help you maintain your focus. If you feel it is appropriate, hang it up in your room, place it on your desk, in your wallet, in your car, or anywhere that will allow you to keep your focus upon it.

HEALING WORDS

The use of healing words or prayer is an excellent way to deal with changes around us that seem beyond our control. For thousands of years prayer has been used as a tool in the healing process. Modern medicine has run scientific tests on the healing power of prayer and the results confirm its effectiveness. Dr Larry Dossey (1993) has compiled an in-depth analysis of research on prayer over the years, and concludes that not only is prayer an effective healing modality but also healing words can be transmitted over huge distances without diminishing their power.

When accounting for how prayer and spiritual practices possibly work to influence health in a local setting, Dossey puts forth many explanations, including the following:

• Belief system precautions regarding hygiene, diet, alcohol, and other *health-related practices* are accepted as being positively associated with health.

• The *social support* involved in group spiritual practices has been documented as a key to health promotion.

• Spiritual faith can be seen in much the same light as the *placebo effect*, with positive expectations resulting in positive outcomes.

The debate between different organizations may always go on as to how to pray, but the research cited in the Dossey volume indicates that directed prayer for a specific well-defined outcome, and non-directed prayer such as "Thy will be done," are both effective.

RECEPTIVE IMAGERY

The techniques described above are powerful tools for healing the body and mind. Another approach is to tune in or become more receptive to what is happening within us that may account for our current state of health and well-being. Receptive imagery is based on the theory that there is an inner intelligence within us that we may be overriding. Using receptive imagery, we can tap into this information, which has been stored in the unconscious mind or perhaps simply ignored in the haste of everyday life.

This technique can be used in conjunction with the progressive deep relaxation to allow us to become more precise in targeting our imagery. It is a simple technique that again requires you to locate yourself in comfortable and quiet surroundings, where you can begin to bring your awareness within. As with the previous techniques, you may want to incorporate it at the end of your progressive deep relaxation session or meditation. It can also be practiced on its own. In the example of stress management, the following approach may be taken. But remember that receptive imagery is equally applicable to all areas of life and health.

EXERCISE

Begin by focusing on the particular area of the body or a particular behavior which attracts stressful reactions. It may be anger or hostility that is accompanied by a raising of the voice and a loss of temper. Use the questions as examples of ways to be receptive to what may be behind your stress. Your answers to the questions will certainly take you into other areas besides those questions listed here, so use these only as a guide:

- *How do you feel when experiencing anger and hostility?*

- *Can you describe the feelings in terms of colors, sounds, or shapes?*

- *Which part of the body do you associate with these colors, sounds, or shapes?*

- *What does this part of the body feel like?*

- *Visualize this area of the body in pictorial form with as much detail as possible.*

- *Familiarize yourself with this mental picture. Get to know it. Acknowledge its existence and ask it how long it has been there.*

- *Ask this picture what its role is.*

- *Does this picture's history and role remind you of any previous experiences in your life?*

- *If so, go back and relive that experience in as much detail as possible.*

- *Now ask that part of the body what it needs to experience physical and emotional healing in order to repair and release the past. Listen carefully.*

- *If you find it is difficult to receive information at this point, imagine a fence or wall. Let it know you appreciate its existence. Ask if it is possible to go beyond it and experience what is on the other side.*

- *Listen and attune to the information that comes forth and be thankful for it.*

- *Thank your inner intelligence for sharing this information and indicate that you would like to facilitate this communication in the future, by discovering the best way to access it.*

Upon completing this receptive imagery technique, write down your experience in your journal and use the information in the other components of this program to help transform yourself. For example, you may become aware of certain feelings and events which have colored the way you are perceiving things and which can be changed in order to experience greater ease. This approach is called reframing, and it is something that we are all capable of doing.

REFRAMING

Through the process of receptive imagery, you may have discovered that you feel you are not good enough in comparison with others. When you reflect on your lifestyle, you may find that you are constantly overindulging in food, work, alcohol, or television as a way to shut out this feeling. Once you have found the source of the problem (in this example, a lack of self-esteem), you can begin to reframe the situation.

Reframing is the ability to look at life from a different perspective. It allows us to change our way of viewing the world and hence our behavior. It is as if we change the glasses we are looking through. If a particular experiment does not work out the way we intended, rather than viewing it as a failure, we give ourselves the credit for trying. The most common illustration of two different perspectives is the

glass filled to midway: is it half full or half empty? If you change
your perspective, you may find that symptoms previously associated
with low self-esteem, such as stress and overeating, disappear of their
own accord.

To reframe, use the HELP tools detailed in this book, and remember
the importance of the stress-reduction techniques from this chapter:

- Take responsibility for stress, realizing that it is not an external
  occurrence.

- Develop an understanding of why stress is occurring (e.g. your
  perspective, expectations).

- Practice techniques that will allow you to transform your
  perspective through:

  —Progressive deep relaxation

  —Guided imagery

  —Positive affirmations

  —Receptive imagery.

And, as with all HELP components, remember to be aware of the
integrated nature of the HELP program and the need to dedicate
yourself to all of its components.

DAILY ROUTINE

Obviously, the more you practice these techniques, the greater the
benefit you will receive. Some of them, such as positive affirmations,
are not time-consuming but require frequent reminders. Other
techniques, such as the guided imagery and receptive imagery, can be
incorporated as part of your daily progressive deep relaxation. The
deep relaxation can be practiced immediately after the yoga postures
(see Chapter 3) for 15 minutes or more. Whenever it is possible to
access these techniques at other times of the day, try to remember
their importance and do them.

HELPFUL HINTS FOR STRESS RELEASE

- Join a yoga class that has a deep relaxation session.

- Use the *Health through Relaxation* audiotape or other guided relaxation tapes.

- Schedule short guided-imagery breaks into your daily routine.

- Get a group of friends together, use the script, and guide one another through deep relaxation.

- Put affirmations in places where you have the most frequent stress responses.

- Take time during the day for prayer.

- Form or join group sessions of healing words or prayer.

FURTHER READING

Benson, Herbert & Klipper, Miriam Z. *The Relaxation Response,* Avon Books, New York, 1976.

Booth, Audrey Livingston. *Stressmanship,* Severn House, London, 1985.

Dossey, Larry. *Healing Words: The Power of Prayer and the Practice of Medicine,* HarperCollins, New York, 1993.

Gawain, Shakti. *Creative Visualization,* Bantam Books, New York, 1979.

Nuernberger, Phil. *Freedom from Stress: A Wholistic Approach,* Himalayan International Institute of Yoga Science, Honesdale, PA, 1981.

Pelletier, Kenneth R. *Mind as Healer, Mind as Slayer,* Delta, New York, 1977.

Selye, Hans. *The Stress of Life,* McGraw-Hill, New York, 1976.

Physical
EXERCISE

AREAS OF HELP IN THIS CHAPTER

Understanding the role of exercise

•

Benefits of exercise

•

Reflecting on physical fitness

•

Body attunement exercise

•

Developing a safe program

•

Components of an exercise routine

•

Weekly schedule

UNDERSTANDING THE ROLE OF EXERCISE

Physical exercise is essential for an easeful body. Conversely, the onset of dis-ease is often due to the fact that our priorities in daily life have not included the development and maintenance of an easeful body. In this chapter you are challenged to determine what your current attitude to the physical body is, attune to the body and its needs, and then learn how to safely improve your physical fitness, and establish a routine that is both practical and enjoyable for you to follow.

To what extent has your awareness of your physical condition been in response to a deterioration of fitness (e.g. restrictions in your ability to move in ways you once were capable of)? Have you engaged in a dynamic process of actively maintaining or improving your overall level of fitness in the absence of any impairments? For most people who are suffering dis-ease of the body, the message they are being sent is one that has existed on a more subtle level for some time. Because they pay so little attention to the body, the message has to be amplified to a level of dis-ability before it attracts their notice.

The process of disease is similar to a situation in which someone is so busy trying to get somewhere that they take no notice of the last time they put fuel in their car. They ignore the gauge on the dashboard because their priorities and mental orientation are elsewhere, and the car still seems to be going. It is only when the car begins to choke, splutter, lurch, and slow down that the message comes through, by which time the car will not take them anywhere until it receives what it needs. Your body has an instruction manual very similar to that of a vehicle, and requires inspection, service, and tuning to prevent it being disabled and out of action. Unfortunately, the stress and distractions of modern life often lead us to toss this manual on a bookshelf somewhere, with good intentions of getting to it once life makes time for it. What choice does the body have in the face of such neglect but to refuse to take us where we want to go unless we attune to its needs?

BENEFITS OF EXERCISE

As a result of our increasingly sedentary lifestyles, as we get older we become more susceptible to arthritis, rheumatism, heart disease, strokes, hypertension, diabetes, persistent or sudden episodes of back pain, and depression. People who have an active fitness plan, combined with the other elements of HELP, can help to reverse this process. You need not be an athlete or sportsperson to experience the benefits of physical activity; a regular program of stretching, walking, and attunement will help you to improve your health without the need for extensive equipment and elaborate training.

The benefits that you will experience include:

- A greater degree of flexibility in the joints of the body

- Increased energy as a result of better circulation, with the blood carrying oxygen to all parts of the body

- Greater strength and cardiovascular fitness as the heart becomes stronger

- Favorable changes in blood cholesterol levels

- Strengthened bones and the prevention of osteoporosis

- Less fatigue as the lungs' efficiency improves

- Increased muscle tone and strength

- Healthier physique as the metabolism is stimulated to assist in burning up fats

- A lift in spirits and outlook as physical activity helps burn biochemicals released by stress and depression and produces endorphins, which relieve pain and elevate emotions

- Improved sleep patterns and relaxation as a result of greater activity

- Facilitated digestion

REFLECTING ON PHYSICAL FITNESS

Take a moment to reflect now on what your attitude has been in recent years to the maintenance and care for your physical fitness. Answer the following questions in your journal and refer back to them as they come up time and again in other chapters:

- Do you have a daily awareness of your level of physical activity?
- Have you set weekly goals or targets that are priorities?
- Can long periods of time slip by without you attending to stretching, exercising, and improving your physical well-being?
- Has this been the case for many years?
- If you were conscious of exercising regularly at one stage of your life, what seem to be the factors associated with the decline in that routine?
- What currently takes precedence over developing a sound approach to physical activity?

Now, in examining the factors that you have listed as taking precedence over physical fitness, can you find any item on the list that you can do well if you are sick? Of course not! It becomes clear immediately when going through this approach that there really are no excuses not to incorporate an active plan for physical exercise, if only so that you are able to carry out your other priorities in life. You cannot attend to the more "pressing matters" of life and ignore your physical fitness, for if you do become ill, you will be unable to attend at all to these matters.

It is time to reacquaint yourself with your body and learn to respect it. Whatever your current state of health, the body has a remarkable capacity to repair and restore itself when you take the time to nurture it. This does require a sensitivity to the needs of the body. A consistent and disciplined approach will complement that sensitivity without you becoming self-absorbed.

BODY ATTUNEMENT EXERCISE

Now take time to attune to the body. In order to develop this sensitivity the following procedure is recommended as a regular practice.

E X E R C I S E

Find a quiet and peaceful place in your home and choose a relaxed time of the day, perhaps early morning before the household or neighbors become active, or in the evening after the day's activities have concluded. Sit in a comfortable and relaxed position, close your eyes, and take in a full and deep breath, following it with a long and relaxed exhalation. Now allow your breathing to follow a deep but relaxed rhythm, and the body to relax with it. Let the mind settle and just be with the breath for a moment.

Ask yourself mentally how the body is feeling at this moment, and scan the body as you visualize the different areas and organs of the body. Is there any part of the body that is sending you subtle signals of tiredness, sluggishness, fatigue, tension, or pain? Take your time to go over the body thoroughly, from the respiratory and digestive systems to the joints and muscles. Experience the body rather than actively thinking about or analyzing it.

Once you have concluded this inner attunement, take a moment to write down any subtle messages you became aware of—both positive and negative. Keep this information as a record in your journal. Record the date and time of each attunement so that you can refer back to it as your body becomes more involved in a disciplined routine, and your awareness is heightened. Record anything and everything that comes up, even if you perceive no signals, either good or bad. This attunement exercise can be done regularly to allow yourself to experience just "being," as well as monitoring the impact of what you are doing.

DEVELOPING A SAFE PROGRAM

Next, you can use this awareness to develop a routine of physical movement that will enhance your overall health. Before embarking on a rigorous program to gain these benefits, you must evaluate your current level of fitness. If you are currently suffering from specific physical ailments such as heart disease, arthritis, respiratory problems, or any major disability, it is always a good idea to clear your proposed fitness program with your health professional. They will be able to evaluate the extent to which the program suits your needs and abilities at this stage.

There are several factors that you should be aware of when developing and carrying out your physical fitness program. The first is the length of time since you last had a regular schedule of physical activity. Keep this in mind when developing your schedule, and build up your capacity slowly if it has been quite some time since you had regular exercise. Always be aware that a gradual daily program which builds up over time as your level of fitness improves is the proper course of action. Avoid intensive programs which once a week tax your system.

Once you have designed an appropriate program, self-monitoring, the second factor, is very important. Begin by discovering your resting pulse rate. To do this follow these steps:

1. Turn one hand over, palm facing upward.

2. Line up the thumb with the index finger, letting it lie on top of it in a straight line.

3. Place the index and middle fingers of the other hand on the thumb and follow its line back to your wrist.

4. There you will find your pulse, on the outer side of the wrist at the base of the thumb.

5. Press down gently and you will feel the pulse beating.

6. Using a watch with a seconds hand, count the beats during a 15-second period and multiply by 4.

A normal pulse rate, depending on age and disease process, will usually fall between 70 and 80 beats per minute. Athletes will have a much slower rate, possibly being as low as 40. The pulse is a very good indicator of the strength of the heart. As you improve your level of fitness, the slower pulse rate will be a sign of a stronger and more efficient heart.

It is important to determine your target heart rate. The maximum heart rate is about 220 beats per minute, but this decreases with age and lack of fitness. Subtract your age from 220 to find your maximum heart rate. When exercising, your pulse should fall in the range of 60 to 75 percent of your maximum heart rate. So, if you are 60 years old, your maximum heart rate is 220–60, or 160. Now multiply 160 by 0.6, which equals 96, and 160 by 0.75, which equals 120. If your pulse rate goes above 120, you are pushing yourself too hard; if it falls below 96, you can exercise more vigorously.

The formula is:

- 220 minus your age for your maximum heart rate (mhr)

- mhr multiplied by 0.6 for the low end of your workout

- mhr multiplied by 0.75 for the high end, which you should not exceed during your fitness regime

Checking your pulse is but one of several indicators which you should keep in mind when working to improve your physical well-being. Evaluate yourself during and after exercise and stretching by asking how the body feels:

- Can you breathe properly while exercising?

- Are you able to talk while exercising?

- Do you feel like you are straining or experiencing pain while carrying out your routine?

Finally, do not hesitate to reduce your routine to one that is challenging but does not go over the fine line into strain and pain. These indicators are there for a reason; do not overrule them hoping they will go away. A slow, enjoyable, regular, and gradual build-up in your capacity is the path to take.

Recent research by Dr Steven Blair confirms that in terms of prolonging life and reducing the chances of disease, a moderate amount of exercise each day, such as walking for 30 minutes per day, will bring almost as much benefit as running 30 to 40 miles (50 to 60 kilometers) a week, when compared to those leading a sedentary lifestyle. So, set realistic and achievable targets that will allow you to keep up a regular practice. Remember, you do not have to run marathons to benefit.

COMPONENTS OF AN EXERCISE ROUTINE

Given the focus on sensitivity to the body and moderation in exercise, your exercise routine should have the following four components: attunement, warm-up phase, continuous rhythmic exercise within your heart range, and cooling-down phase. All four components are equally important and none should be neglected or rushed.

Attunement

The attunement exercise is the beginning of the routine and involves two minutes of withdrawing your awareness from external distractions such as sounds, other people, smells, and visual objects. Just close the eyes and focus on the breath. Then scan the body and alert yourself to any subtle signals the body may be trying to communicate to you before you engage in your exercise routine. By doing this practice regularly, you can develop your awareness of the internal intelligence of the body and trigger a greater sensitivity to it in order to avoid strain or injury. If a symptom comes up, do not dismiss it but keep it in your awareness so as not to overtax that part of the body during your routine. Mentally try to visualize that part of the body and release any tension or stiffness by relaxing the area and breathing in slowly and deeply. If the symptom persists or gets worse, it will be necessary to explore what may be causing it more actively and perhaps seek the advice of a health professional. By attuning to these signals on a subtle level, we can often avoid injury.

Warm-up Phase

The warm-up phase of activity is an essential part of your routine and should last for about 10 minutes. The benefits include:

- Preparing the cardiovascular system and the respiratory system for exercise

- Increasing flexibility of the body

- Slowly increasing body temperature

- Helping to avoid muscle strains

The ideal sequence is to warm the body up and then do some gentle stretching to avoid injuring cold muscles. Your warm-up can be as simple as slowly jogging in place, using a stationary cycle, or a gentle rehearsal of the sport or exercise you're about to perform.

Next begin to stretch the muscles and move the joints slowly. A series of stretches that are suitable for both the warm-up and cool-down phases follow. Also feel free to incorporate any of the yoga postures included in the easeful body chapter that you may find useful. The yoga postures are excellent for both warm-up and cool-down stretches as they involve:

• Stretching and toning of muscles

• Flexibility of joints

• Mindfulness of the body

• Awareness of feelings

• Proper posture

• Slow and easeful movements

Limbering up the Body

Stretching the joints of the body is a great place to begin, and with all movement the awareness should be with the stretch and the breathing, keeping that inner attunement as you move.

E X E R C I S E

Foot and Leg Stretches

Begin by sitting down on the floor with your legs stretched out in front of you. Bring your awareness to the toes of each foot and begin moving the toes backward and forward, first with the right foot and then with the left, for 20 seconds each foot.

Begin to stretch and loosen the ankles by rotating one foot at a time in a circular clockwise direction for 10 seconds, then anticlockwise for 10 seconds.

Next, keeping the left leg stretched out, bend the right leg and place the right foot on top of the left knee or thigh (or, if not possible, on the inside of the left leg). Begin to lift up the right knee, then slowly lower it as far as you can without straining. You may want to use the right hand to help the knee come down further. Continue raising and lowering for 20 seconds. Now release the right leg and reverse sides, bending the left knee and placing the left foot in position on the right leg, and again raising up and lowering down for 20 seconds.

With the soles of the feet together, bring the feet as close to the groin area as is comfortable and slowly raise the knees up and down, feeling free to use the hands or the elbows to help the knees go down in the direction of the floor without straining. Continue for 30 seconds.

Hand and Arm Stretches

Continue sitting on the floor. Extend your right arm out in front of you, splay out the fingers of the right hand, then make a fist. Continue expanding and contracting the hand for 20 seconds, then begin with the left hand.

Now stretch the right wrist by rotating the hand in a clockwise direction for 20 seconds, then anticlockwise for 20 seconds. Follow with the left wrist and hand.

For the elbow, upper arm and shoulder joints, stretch the right arm high above the head, reaching up toward the sky and splaying the fingers as you stretch upward. Now bend the elbow and lower the hand down to the top of the shoulder. Repeat 10 times, then relax the right arm and begin with the left.

Combined Leg and Arm Stretches

Lie on your back, with your arms extending above your head on the floor and your legs stretched out in front of you. Extend your limbs out in opposite directions, stretching the arms past the head, and the legs and feet in the opposite direction. Hold for 5 seconds, then relax for a few seconds and stretch out once more.

Next bend the right leg and, keeping the left leg straight, clasp your hands just below the right knee and help the right knee down to the chest area as you compress the abdomen muscles. Hold while you slowly raise your head toward the right knee. Hold for a count of three, then lower the head down, release the hands, lower the right leg down and relax for 10 seconds. Reverse the process with the left leg.

After resting, bring up both knees toward the chest, wrap your arms just below the knees and bring the knees down toward the chest. Hold for 3 seconds with the option of lifting up the head in the direction of the knees.

Upper Back, Shoulder, and Neck Stretches

Remember never to strain the neck muscles—always start slowly. Come up to a standing position with the feet about shoulder width apart and the arms stretched out to the sides in a T shape. Slowly swing from side to side, rotating from the waist. When you rotate to the left, swing the right hand toward the left shoulder giving yourself a pat on the back; and on the other side, swing the left hand toward the right shoulder. Continue for 30 seconds increasing the speed moderately. Allow the head and neck to swing gently further and further back, looking over the shoulder you are swinging to, but without straining the neck. Feel the spine and back area loosen up with the stretch. When concluding, slow down the movements gently, returning to the standing position, and allow the breath to return to normal.

Next, raise the shoulders toward the ears and hold to a count of 5, then exhale and allow the shoulders to lower. Continue with shoulder shrugs for three rounds. Then, keeping the head facing forward, lower the head in the direction of the right shoulder, hold for 10 seconds, then slowly raise the head back up to center. Lower the head down to the left shoulder and hold for 10 seconds. Center the head and relax. Remember always to be gentle with the neck.

Lower Back and Hamstrings

Have the feet together and the knees slightly bent in a standing position as you slowly bend forward from the hips, keeping the back straight. Allow your arms to stretch down toward the floor until you feel your hamstrings and back muscles stretch. Keep the knees bent, and do not bounce or use force to try to reach the floor. Hold for 20 seconds, then slowly come up and relax.

Continuous Rhythmic Exercise

Once the body is loose and warmed up, it is appropriate to begin the aerobic portion of the fitness routine, with the type of activity being governed by your:

• Current level of fitness

• Ability to access this activity on a regular basis

• Particular interests or inclination

When previously engaged in physical activity years ago you might have been a marathon runner, but of course it would be dangerous to go back to that immediately after years of a sedentary lifestyle. Similarly, you may choose cross-country skiing as the activity you would most like to do, but unless you have access to it regularly you will need to find other activities to incorporate. Finally, if you choose an activity such as swimming but you do not enjoy it, there is little chance that your fitness program will be successful. Remember the three As of aerobic exercise: **Appropriate, Accessible, Agreeable.**

Appropriate Exercise

The distinction between aerobic exercise and anaerobic exercise is an important one to remember. Anaerobic exercise, such as weight lifting and sit-ups, involves short bursts of activity, and burns glucose (sugar) stored within the muscle for fuel. It helps to build muscular strength but has limited benefits for the cardiorespiratory system and does not lead to fat loss. Aerobic exercise, such as walking, swimming, and jogging, involves continuous rhythmic movement over an extended period of time, and uses oxygen for fuel. Aerobic exercise benefits the cardiorespiratory system and leads to fat loss, as the muscles burn a percentage of fat for fuel. While both activities are beneficial, it is important to ensure that you incorporate aerobic exercise into your routine.

To determine whether your aerobic activities are appropriate, they should meet the following criteria:

• If you have not exercised for a long time, are under medical supervision, or are suffering from a disability, you should consult with your health-care professional.

- Your chosen activity should meet the four conditions of the FITT principle, which are frequency, intensity, time, and type of exercise:
Frequency (how often to exercise)—This will obviously vary according to your level of fitness and the type of activity chosen, but should eventually be three to five times per week.
Intensity (how hard to exercise)—The exercise should fall within the pulse rate range, which you calculated as being between 60 and 75 percent of your maximum pulse rate.
Time (how long to exercise)—The exercise should be sustained for 20 to 60 minutes, depending on frequency.
Type (what type of exercise)—The exercise should involve continuous rhythmic movement of large muscle groups, and such activities as walking, jogging, aerobic dance, bicycling, swimming, and rowing are all suitable.

- You should experience no unusual symptoms, during or after exercise, such as extreme shortness of breath after mild exertion, dizziness, fainting, nausea, cold sweating, confusion, pain or pressing in the chest, neck, shoulders, arms, throat or jaw, or abnormal heart activity such as an irregular heart rhythm.

Accessible Exercise

The importance of accessibility should not be minimized, as it will have a great deal of impact on the success of your program. To determine the accessibility of your chosen activity, answer the following questions:

- Is the cost of the activity within your present budget and within budgets of the foreseeable future?

- Can you easily get to the activity without being reliant on things out of your personal control?

- Do you need a partner for this activity and, if so, is one likely to be readily available all the time?

- If there is special equipment needed for this activity, is it available and affordable?

- Is this activity dependent on the weather, and what alternatives do you have in case of unpleasant weather?

- Do you have the required skill level to perform this activity at present?

- Does the time of day suitable for this activity fit in with your other responsibilities?

By answering these questions honestly, you will be able to choose an activity or two which are likely to work for you.

Agreeable Exercise

Once you have one or more activities that meet the first two requirements of being appropriate and accessible, choose activities that are agreeable to you and that you will enjoy. In terms of motivating yourself to exercise regularly, this last factor is particularly important as you will not stick to a fitness regimen that you dislike. You may prefer:

- A variety of activities that will allow you to remain stimulated and not get in a rut

- Activities that bring you into contact with other people who can help you stay motivated and provide a pleasant atmosphere

- Activities that challenge you in terms of skill development

- Activities that will leave you feeling good about yourself and your accomplishments

- Activities that have secondary benefits other than the aerobic value, such as taking you out into nature, or bringing you into contact with old friends or a pleasant and stimulating environment

Commitment

Once you have chosen the activities that you feel satisfy the three As, follow these suggestions in order to make a commitment to your exercise routine:

- Keep a record of your goals, setting small weekly goals as a first step and building up to your long-term goals.

- Remind yourself that you owe it to yourself to maintain your fitness. Let some people know your intended program and ask them to assist you in keeping your commitment.

- Enter details of your progress, any problems, lapses, thoughts, and feelings into your journal.

- Reward yourself when you have met your goals, acknowledging your effort.

- If for circumstances beyond your control you have had a setback, do not let that affect your commitment. Whatever the cause of your lapse, get going again.

- Remind yourself of the benefits, which include more energy, greater resistance to illness and stress, stronger bones, stronger heart and respiratory system, better self-image, and increased confidence.

Cooling-down Phase

When concluding your aerobic activity, it is essential to allow the body time to cool down for a period of five to ten minutes. By developing a routine for cooling down after exertion, you can avoid muscle soreness, allow your pulse to slowly return to the resting rate, and enjoy the winding-down process after your workout. If you just stopped moving after exercising, the heart would still be beating rapidly without sufficient blood returning to it.

The cooling-down approach should first consist of reducing the speed gradually of the aerobic activity you are engaged in, slowing it right down. This can then be followed by some of the warm-up stretches illustrated previously, which are suitable for both limbering up the body and cooling it down. Just take them slowly and with awareness, letting the muscles relax into them and the heart slow down. These stretches as well as some of the yoga postures in Chapter 3 will provide a good transition for the muscles and joints to adjust to the decline of physical exertion, and reduce the chances of musculoskeletal injury.

WEEKLY SCHEDULE

When planning your weekly schedule take into consideration the following factors:

- After seeking advice from your health professional (if necessary in your case), set achievable goals. Even if it means you will not be meeting the goal of three hours of aerobic exercise per week immediately, try to work up to that with either six 30-minute sessions or three one-hour sessions per week.

- Plan out your weekly program, taking into consideration other HELP components, including stress-management techniques.

- Come up with a schedule that is realistic for you, given your other responsibilities, and then commit yourself to it.

- If after some time it becomes apparent that you are capable of doing more, be gradual in your approach, remembering that it is far better to be consistent in a schedule that may be slightly below your capability than to push yourself to 100 percent inconsistently, with stress.

- No matter what activity you have chosen, make a commitment to it, monitor yourself, evaluate the schedule, and remind yourself of the benefits of regular exercise and the goals you have set.

HELPFUL HINTS FOR PHYSICAL EXERCISE

- Join or establish an exercise group.

- Exercise to raise funds for a charity.

- Reward yourself for meeting your exercise goals.

- Combine exercise with getting out into nature.

- Variety is the spice of exercise.

FURTHER READING

American College of Sports Medicine. *ACSM Fitness Book,* Human Kinetics Publishers, Champaign, IL, 1992.

Anderson, Bob. *Stretching,* Shelter Publications, Bolinas, CA, 1980.

Blair, SN et al. "Physical Fitness and All Cause Mortality," *Journal of American Medical Association,* 262, 1989, 2395-2401.

Tobias, Maxine & Sullivan, John Patrick. *Complete Stretching,* Knopf, New York, 1992.

Wicks, John. *Guide to Exercise,* National Heart Foundation of Australia, Melbourne, 1983.

An Easeful BODY

AREAS OF HELP IN THIS CHAPTER

Understanding easefulness

·

Reflecting on daily activities

·

Benefits of yoga

·

Preparing for hatha yoga

·

A yoga routine

·

Massage

·

Daily routine

UNDERSTANDING EASEFULNESS

When examining the linkages between our lifestyles and overall well-being, the two primary areas of exploration are the mind and the body. Previously we explored the relationship between aerobic exercise and health, with the key being continuous rhythmic movement within your range of safety. This chapter is designed to bring even greater awareness of the physical body through yoga. As we begin to attune to the physical body through yoga postures, we will gain a deeper understanding of lifestyle factors that may need to be developed to promote a more harmonious body/mind dynamic.

The body is the grounding or physical expression of our genetic make-up, our lifestyle patterns, our thoughts and emotions, and our outlook on life. Through gaining a greater awareness of the physical body we can attune to the factors that may be underlying our current state of ease or dis-ease. By stretching, moving, listening to the body, and beginning to look after it, we can also find that our thoughts, emotions, lifestyle, and outlook on life are directly benefited. As neuromessengers are released through our mental activities, so too with physical stretching of the body are hormones and chemicals released into the body which then leave us feeling healthier and happier.

Working on mental enhancement but ignoring the body is like building a beautiful house without taking adequate time to establish a solid foundation, and this is reflected in many age-old sayings: "A healthy mind is a healthy body," "The body is the temple of the soul," "An easeful body, a peaceful mind, and a useful life." It is important to reacquaint ourselves with the body, attune to its needs, and begin to remedy blockages that exist through a regular routine of stretching. If we learn to look after the body and to listen to it, the quality of our life will improve beyond the time and energy we have spent on making the body easeful.

Our bodies reflect the stress and strain of daily concerns through the tensing and contracting of muscles. Whether it is because of a clenched jaw, or stiffness and tension in the shoulders and neck, we are all aware of feeling less than easeful at times. This is not necessarily a result of physical straining but may be from our thoughts, feelings, and situations we find ourselves in that we perceive as stressful.

Learning to stretch the body, attune to it, and lengthen muscles that are chronically tight as a result of stress will help to rebalance both the body and the mind. As the body loosens up, physiological changes will be taking place to allow the mind to benefit from this as well. Researchers have found that when people are asked to perform different simple movements (e.g. smiling, frowning), their bodies respond with physiological changes in areas such as breathing and heart rate. The body is not just a reflection of our thoughts and emotions; there is an interactive dynamic that also allows our physical expression and movement to affect our mental state of well-being.

REFLECTING ON DAILY ACTIVITIES

Take a moment to reflect upon your weekly schedule. Relax by scanning your body mentally and releasing any tension. Think about your activities over a typical week. Ask yourself whether your body is becoming more flexible and supple as a result of these activities. Focus on specific regions—shoulders, neck, lower back, spine, knees, feet—and become aware of any muscular tension or stiffness in these areas. Do your daily activities enhance coordination, range of movement, and strength of the body? When you are ready, take out your journal and answer the following questions:

- On average, how many total hours a day do you spend sitting at a desk, in the car, at meals, or relaxing?

- How many hours do you spend sleeping?

- How much time do you spend exerting yourself through physical exercise?

- How much time do you spend slowly stretching the body for greater flexibility?

The answers to these questions will serve as a starting point for the development of a more easeful body. It is common for most people to spend a great deal of time sitting or sleeping, doing only limited physical exercise, and very little if any stretching. As a result, areas of the body can become stiff and painful, with a limited range of movement. Disease, poor blood circulation, and muscular weakness are commonly associated with this sedentary lifestyle. Simple movements that once were relatively easy—bending, lifting, twisting—become restricted. Organs of the body malfunction. Arthritis and muscular aches and pains can set in.

Through this reflection you may find that it is time to address these areas by incorporating a regular routine to regain an easeful body. Hatha yoga postures have been used for thousands of years to develop and maintain a flexible and healthy body, leading to a more peaceful mind and useful life.

BENEFITS OF YOGA

Hatha yoga is a system of stretching the body that encourages awareness, is non competitive, is accessible to everyone, does not require endurance, is open to modification based on level of flexibility, reduces stress, requires no equipment purchase, and has been developed over thousands of years. The stretching postures work on the spine, making it supple and healthy, and thus promoting the maximum fresh blood supply to all the organs, glands, and tissues. By the gentle pressure of the postures the endocrine glands are toned, which results in both physical and psychological benefits.

Some other benefits of regular hatha yoga practice include the maintaining and restoring of:

• Muscle strength and resilience

• Neuromuscular coordination

• Exercise tolerance

• Normal bowel function with regular elimination

• Musculoskeletal flexibility and joint range of movement

- Circulatory and respiratory efficiency including cardiac output, return of blood to the heart, and blood oxygenation

- Bone strength and structural integrity of joints

- Healthy lipid and cholesterol metabolism

- Sensitivity to insulin with resultant enhanced glucose metabolism

- Ability to respond constructively to challenges and stress

- Immune function, replacement of red and white blood cells

PREPARING FOR HATHA YOGA

It is clear that the benefits of the yoga postures are numerous as long as there is regularity of practice with awareness not to strain in any of the postures. These postures are meant to be flowing, not bouncing, and done with a sense of inner attunement. When doing the postures, try to keep the mind centered on the breath and the stretch. Avoid getting caught up in mental distractions by always returning to the breathing.

If you have any injuries or health ailments, please go over this routine with your health practitioner before starting.

When preparing for your session:

- Wear comfortable, loose-fitting clothing that will not restrain your stretching in any way.

- Remove any jewelry or objects that may get in the way.

- Choose a location that is suitable in the sense that it is peaceful, clean, with good ventilation, carpeted if possible, and quiet.

- Lay out a mat, towel, blanket, or sheet on which to do your practices.

- If you have an old injury or are in any way concerned with your ability to do the postures, be sure to discuss these concerns beforehand with your health professional to see if they need to be modified in any way.

The key with all the postures is to do them within your own range of

flexibility. Remember that this is not an endurance test or
competition, and the body must remain steady and comfortable in
each posture. If you feel the body trembling, if the breath is forced, or
if you feel like you are pushing yourself beyond the range of comfort,
it is time to come out of the pose and relax. Be sure to leave time in
between the postures for the body and breath to relax. It is
recommended that women suspend practice of the shoulder stand
during time of menstruation.

E X E R C I S E

A YOGA ROUTINE

*The routine illustrated here was brought to the West by Sri Swami
Satchidananda, and is taught as part of Integral Yoga.*

*It is a good idea to begin your practice by sitting for a moment with
your eyes closed, and scanning the body. As you pass from the feet,
gradually moving from part to part up to the head, mentally release
any tension from the body. Become in touch with the body and how you
feel at this point. Take this time to begin to bring the awareness within:
let go of external sounds, sights, and smells, and focus your mind on
internal sensations. Start with a full deep inhalation followed by a long
relaxed exhalation, and repeat this deep breath twice.*

*It is also important to stretch and limber up the body with the sun
salutation, which acts as a warm-up and general tonic for the entire
system. A word about breathing: once you have learned the
movements, aim to breathe smoothly in and out throughout the
duration of each position. Eventually you may allow the pace to flow
with no hesitation between each position. The whole sun salutation
becomes one continuous movement.*

*Repeat this series of movements two or three times. The tempo can be slow
if you feel agitated or you can do the movements more rapidly if you
want it to alert the mind and invigorate the body to relieve sluggishness.*

Benefits: Improves and maintains flexibility. A general tonic for the
entire system. Excellent for depression.

Sun Salutation or the 12-Part Movement

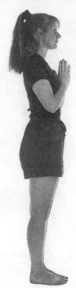

FIGURE 3.1 *Position 1: Exhale. Stand up straight with your feet together.*
Bring your palms together in front of your chest.

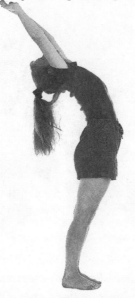

FIGURE 3.1 *Position 2: Inhale. Lock your thumbs. Stretch out your arms in*
front of you. Watch your hands as you slowly raise your arms overhead.
Bend backward a little from the hips as you stretch.

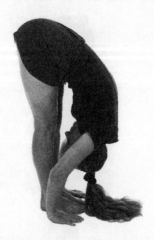

FIGURE 3.1 Position 3: Exhale. Fold forward from the hips as you stretch out and then down toward the floor, keeping the knees straight. Look back down toward the knees as the hands stretch down in the direction of the floor.

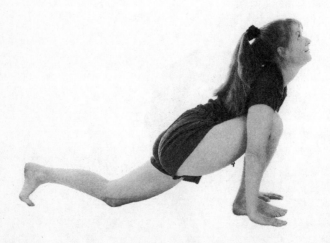

FIGURE 3.1 Position 4: Inhale. Bend your knees and place your palms alongside your feet with the fingertips and toes in a straight line. Stretch your left leg back, placing your left knee on the floor. Leave your right foot between your hands and bring your right knee to your chest. Look up.

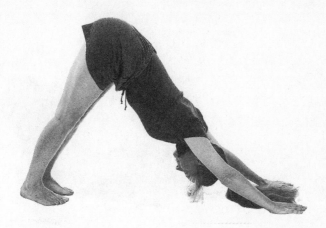

FIGURE 3.1 *Position 5: Exhale. Take your right foot back to meet your left. Raise your buttocks so that your body now forms a triangle. Stretch your heels toward the floor and look at your feet.*

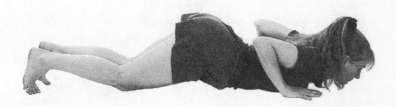

FIGURE 3.1 *Position 6: Begin to inhale. Lower your knees, then chest and chin to the floor, leaving your pelvis slightly raised. Your palms are now beneath your shoulders, your elbows close to your body and pointing upward.*

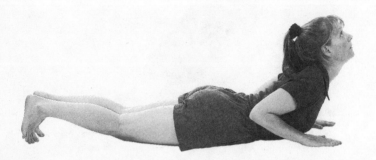

FIGURE 3.1 *Position 7: Continue to inhale as you lower your pelvis to the floor. Stretch up your head, neck, and chest. Keep your elbows slightly bent and in toward your body.*

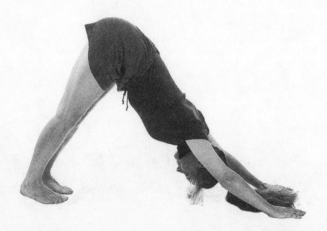

FIGURE 3.1 *Position 8: Exhale. Press down on your palms and feet to lift your buttocks, forming a triangle as before, with heels pressing down and head looking to feet.*

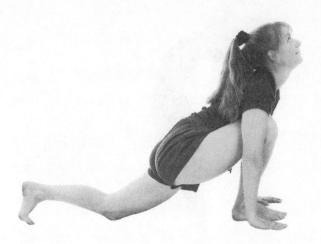

FIGURE 3.1 *Position 9: Inhale. Move your left foot forward between your hands, with your left knee touching your chest. The right leg is now stretched back, with your right knee on the floor. Look up.*

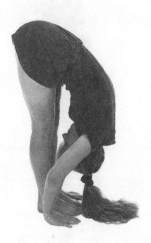

FIGURE 3.1 *Position 10: Exhale. Bring your right foot forward to meet the left. Bring your feet together and straighten your knees as you stretch down, as though touching your toes. Bend from your hips only as far as you feel comfortable. Head looking back to the knees.*

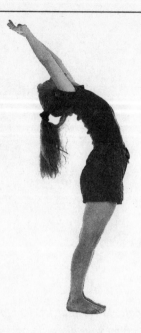

FIGURE 3.1 *Position 11: Inhale. Again lock your thumbs, stretch out toward the center and up toward the ceiling, and bend backward slightly as in position 2. Looking at the hands.*

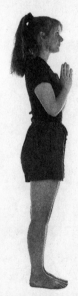

FIGURE 3.1 *Position 12: Exhale. Slowly bring your palms together in front of your chest. Relax.*

Back Stretch (Cobra Pose)

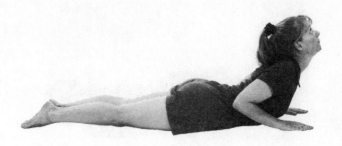

FIGURE 3.2

Lie on your abdomen. Place your palms on the floor beneath your shoulders, with your fingers pointing forward and your elbows raised and close to your body, as if you were going to do a push-up. Keep your legs together and your toes pointed.

Inhale. Stretch your chin forward and, without pushing down on your hands, slowly raise your head, then neck, then chest off the floor. Keep your pelvis on the floor, and try not to place any weight on your hands. Breathe normally.

At the beginning, hold this position for only a few seconds, repeating it twice. Exhale as you slowly roll down, first touching your chin, then your forehead to the ground. Turn your cheek to the side but leave your hands in place, and relax. At your own pace, gradually increase the time you spend in this position (up to a minute) and do it fewer times. The last time you come down, turn your cheek to the side, release your arms and legs, allowing the arms to rest alongside the torso, and spend a few seconds in the resting position on your abdomen.

Benefits: Excellent stretch for spine, back muscles, cranial nerves. Releases tension and aches from back and neck. Opens chest cavity, relieves constipation and gas.

Leg Lift One (Half Locust Pose)

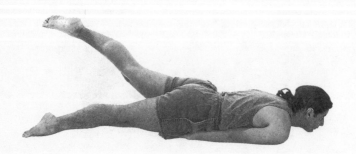

FIGURE 3.3

Lie facedown with your chin on the ground. Push your arms underneath your body, with your elbows close under your body and your palms facing your thighs. Keep your pelvis on your arms.

Inhale, straighten your right leg, then slowly raise it off the floor as far as you feel comfortable. Hold it in the air for up to 10 seconds while breathing normally, then slowly lower it down. Repeat with your left leg.

Do this twice with each leg.

Benefits: Excellent stretch for back, abdomen, pelvis.

Leg Lift Two (Full Locust Pose)

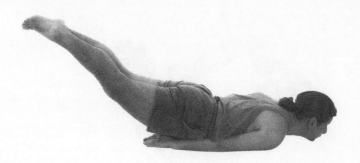

FIGURE 3.4

As shown, inhale, but this time stiffen the body, keep your chin on the floor, and raise both legs together a comfortable distance without bending your knees. Try to keep knees together and feet together. Breathe normally.

Repeat twice, holding for up to 10 seconds each time.

Benefits: Same as above. Also tones the sympathetic nervous system, improves liver function, and relieves the pain of lumbago.

Backward Bend (Bow Pose)

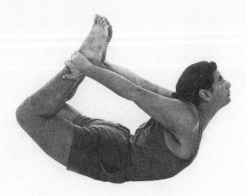

FIGURE 3.5

Lie facedown. Bend the knees and bring the heels toward the buttocks. Reach and grasp the ankles or feet. Bring the forehead to the floor. Raise the head, then the chest and thighs, arching the back to allow the weight to balance on the abdomen. Keep the arms straight, the knees can be apart, and the awareness is on the entire spine. Come out of the pose in the reverse order. This is not to be practiced by those with a stomach or intestinal ulcer, or with high blood pressure or a hernia.

Benefits: Reduces abdominal fat and increases peristalsis of the bowels.

Forward Stretch One (Head-to-Knee Pose)

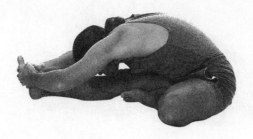

FIGURE 3.6

Sit on the floor and stretch out both of your legs in front of you. Bend your left leg and place the sole of your left foot on the inside of your right knee or thigh if you can.

Inhale, look up, lock your thumbs, and raise your arms overhead as far as you comfortably can.

Exhale, bending forward from the hips and keeping your back straight. Stretch out over the right leg as far as you feel comfortable. Then take hold of your right foot, calf, or whatever you can comfortably reach. Allow your head to relax. Breathe normally.

Hold this position for up to 10 seconds, then repeat with your other leg. Repeat two or three times with each leg. With regular practice, gradually increase the time you can spend in this position and do it fewer times. Then relax on the back.

Benefits: Tones abdominal organs, activates kidneys, liver, pancreas, and adrenal glands. Stretches hamstrings and loosens the hip joints.

Forward Stretch Two (Forward Bending Pose)

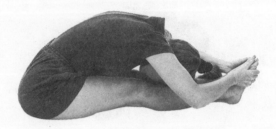

FIGURE 3.7

This pose is the same as the head-to-knee pose, but instead of bending one leg, you stretch out over both legs together.

Stretch your arms up over your head, sitting firmly on your buttocks, back and neck straight. Then, folding forward from the hips, stretch out over both legs first. Once you have extended as far forward as feels comfortable, slowly lower your hands down on the feet or legs, allowing the head, neck, and shoulders to relax.

If you want to go deeper into the pose, raise the upper body with an inhalation, and, as you exhale, extend further out over the legs and lower down.

Repeat twice, holding for 10 seconds. Gradually increase the time in the pose (up to 30 seconds) and come into it just once as you become more comfortable with it through regular practice.

Benefits: Stretches back and buttock muscles. Excellent for the bladder, prostate, and lumbar nerves.

Shoulder Stand (Modified I & II)

Do only these modified versions if you have high blood pressure, neck or shoulder injuries, back pain, or if you have had problems with the other postures.

Modified I: Lie on your back and elevate your legs by resting your feet on a chair seat. Maintain this position for two or three minutes, less if you become uncomfortable.

Benefits: Excellent for the blood circulation.

Modified II: If you have none of these challenges and would like to go one step further, allow your calf muscles to also rest on the chair seat then, grasping hold of the chair seat with both hands, place the feet on the top of the back support of the chair allowing your thighs or buttocks to be supported fully by the front edge of the chair seat with both hands holding the chair seat firmly. If comfortable, tuck the chin into the chest and lift the feet off the back of the chair with the knees as straight as possible. Breathe normally. Hold only as long as you feel steady and comfortable. When you are ready to come down,

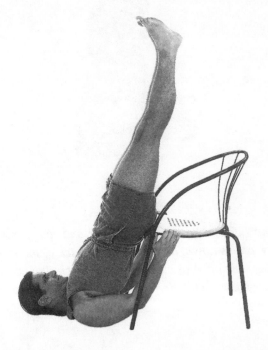

FIGURE 3.8

slowly lower your legs back onto the chair, then place your feet on the seat with your buttocks returning to the floor. Lower the legs back to the floor releasing your hands from the chair and roll over onto one shoulder. Then sit for a moment to regain your balance. Avoid doing inverted postures during time of menstruation.

Shoulder Stand (Regular)

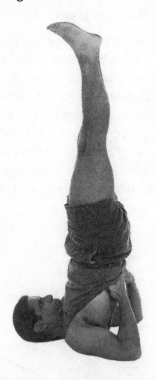

FIGURE 3.9

Lie on your back with your feet together and your arms alongside your body, palms down. Be aware of the back of the neck area and remove any hair or obstacles behind the neck. Try not to cough, swallow, or sneeze while in the pose; if you need to do so, come out of the pose in the reverse order.

Inhale, straighten your legs and lift them up to a 90-degree angle. Press on the palms and swing the legs slightly overhead or parallel to the floor and bring the hands to your lower back for support. (You may find that you need to bend the knees in order to raise your legs over your head.) Gradually straighten your legs to a vertical position, bringing your chin and chest close together. Breathe normally. Hold for only as long as you feel comfortable and steady, feeling free to reposition the hands, bringing them closer to the spine and further down toward the shoulder blades to give you more support and to keep you straight.

When you are ready, slowly lower your legs over your head again so that they are parallel to the floor, transfer your forearms to the floor, bring your trunk down slowly, then lower your legs slowly to the ground. If your abdomen is not strong enough to allow this, just roll down slowly with control, in whatever way is most comfortable for you.

Benefits: Excellent for the circulatory, digestive, and nervous systems. Stimulates the thyroid gland, helping to regulate the body's metabolism.

Chest Extension (Fish Pose)

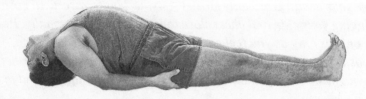

FIGURE 3.10

Lie on your back. Bring your legs together and grasp the sides of your thighs. Resting your weight on your elbows, raise your head and trunk to a half-seated position. Arch your back, thrusting out your chest. Lower your head and place the top of your head on the floor. Your weight should be balanced between the top of your head, your elbows, and your buttocks. Have a slight smile on your face to relax any tension in your jaw. Hold for one-third of the time that you held the shoulder stand.

To come down, shift your weight to your elbows, straighten your neck and back, then slowly lower to the floor. Whenever you do the shoulder stand, always follow it with the fish pose as it helps to balance the shoulder stand.

Benefits: Opens up the chest cavity and oxygenates the lungs. Useful for people suffering from asthma or bronchitis. Massages neck and shoulders. Excellent for improving posture.

Half Spinal Twist

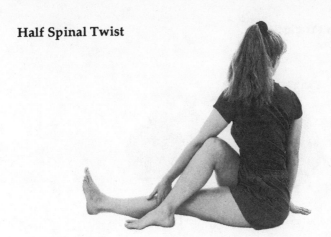

FIGURE 3.11

*Sit on the floor and extend your left leg straight out in front of you.
Cross your right foot over your left knee, placing the sole of your
right foot flat on the floor. Sit up straight. Bring your right knee close
to your chest. Now extend your arms in front of you, lock your thumbs
and twist to the right.*

*Unlock your thumbs and place your right hand on the floor behind
you, close to your body, with your fingers pointing away from you.
Place your left arm between your trunk and your right knee (on the
outside of your right knee), and press your knee to the right.*

*Reach around your right knee with your left hand and take hold of the
outside of your left leg or the instep of your right foot. Slowly twist
your head and trunk to the right and look over your right shoulder.
After 15 to 60 seconds, slowly unwind and do the same pose on the
other side.*

Benefits: Excellent for liver, spleen, kidneys, and adrenal glands.
Strengthens the back muscles.

Forward Stretch (Yogic Seal)

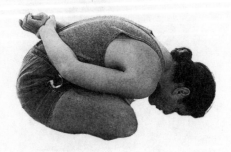

FIGURE 3.12

Sit in a comfortable seated position with your legs crossed and eyes closed. Take both hands behind your back and grasp your right wrist with your left hand. Sit up straight and inhale deeply.

Exhale, bending forward from your hips. Come forward as far as is comfortable and allow the head to lower and with practice rest on the floor. You may wish to spend several minutes relaxing into the position, letting go of tension in your neck, back, and shoulders.

To come out of the pose, extend your chin, inhale, then return to a seated position, keeping the back straight, and release the hands. Just sit for a moment with the eyes closed feeling the balancing effect.

Benefits: Massages the abdominal organs. Tones the entire nervous system.

MASSAGE

Another useful tool for improving flexibility and relieving muscular distress is massage. Through massage you can release tension that may have been stored in specific areas of the body for years. While the variety of massage techniques available may seem a bit confusing at first, it is just a matter of experiencing what feels comfortable for you. A complete deep body massage provides the following benefits on a physiological level:

- Improves muscle tone

- Increases the flow of nutrients to the muscles

- Cleanses the body of toxins by promoting the flow of lymph

- Dilates the blood vessels and promotes circulation

- Relieves muscle tension

In addition to providing numerous physical benefits, massage works on a psychological level. Through releasing tension, you begin to feel more comfortable with your body. This in turn promotes a more joyful and peaceful approach to life.

DAILY ROUTINE

When doing the hatha yoga postures you should allot at least 20 minutes, in combination with the other practices that follow, to go through the series of movements. Look over your schedule and determine the best time of the day for you to do these practices regularly. Morning is ideal as hatha yoga is a great way to start the day and if for some reason you cannot do it, you still have the rest of the day to fit it in. Never take the attitude that it is all or nothing. Even if on a particularly busy day you have only a few minutes to spend on stretching, it is far better to do a few sun salutations than nothing at all.

Know that it is through regular practice, with a sense of commitment and inner attunement, that the benefits discussed earlier will come. Do not compare yourself with others. *Remember never to strain.* Be accepting of where you are at each moment with no judgment as to progress being made. Your daily schedule will ensure that over time the body will derive all the benefits of these movements, and the mind will become increasingly peaceful.

If you choose to hold postures for longer periods of time as you become more flexible, ensure that you do not eliminate part of your routine, as each pose balances the next and provides a particular benefit. Also, if you hold the postures for longer periods of time and increase the overall time of your routine, do not reduce the time dedicated to other components of the program. The integrated nature of HELP is crucial to its effectiveness.

HELPFUL HINTS FOR AN EASEFUL BODY

- Join a yoga class.

- Use a HELP audiotape or video to guide you through the yoga routine.

- Try other methods of gentle stretching such as tai chi or qi gong.

- Have massages to keep the body supple.

- Participate in a yoga retreat.

FURTHER READING

Mandelkorn, Philip (ed). *To Know Your Self: The Essential Teachings of Swami Satchidananda,* Integral Yoga Publications, Buckingham, Virginia, 1978.

Saraswati, Satyananda. *Asana, Pranayama, Mudra,* Bandha, Bihar School of Yoga, Monghyr, Bihar, India, 1977.

Satchidananda, Swami. *Integral Yoga Hatha,* Holt, Rinehart & Winston, New York, 1975.

Schatz, Mary Pulig. Article in *Yoga Journal,* May/June 1990,

Sivananda, Swami. *Health and Hatha Yoga,* Divine Life Society, Sivanandanagar, India, 1985.

$\mathcal{A}$ $\mathcal{Q}$uality
ENVIRONMENT

—

AREAS OF **HELP** IN THIS CHAPTER

Understanding environmental influences

•

Reflecting on our environments

•

Creating a quality environment

•

Simple tips for fine-tuning the workplace

•

Weekly schedule

UNDERSTANDING ENVIRONMENTAL INFLUENCES

We have all noticed the impact that walking into a beautiful garden—with its lushness, fragrance, color array, bird sounds, butterflies, dynamism, and vitality—has on our sense of well-being. Likewise, we can all recall entering a building that prompted us to look for an immediate way out, given its lack of fresh air, monotony of tones, stale smells, haphazardness, noise, and low energy. Upon entering any setting our senses immediately send us direct feedback on all levels. The environment can set the tone of our emotions—whether we feel comfortable or tense, excited or lethargic, healthy or claustrophobic, friendly or stiff, involved or aloof—and therefore it conditions us in many ways of which we may not even be aware. This chapter is about understanding what a quality environment means to us, and how to create one that will promote a healthy lifestyle.

Given human differences and the diverse nature of the world around us, it cannot be assumed that everyone agrees on what constitutes a quality environment. Rather than trying to detail specific objects or a specific design that you should include in your workplace, for example, this chapter is all about general guidelines to be aware of when designing your own quality environment. The notion of taking the time to reflect on your present environment and whether it is conducive to a healthy lifestyle is the key to this component of HELP.

Just as our mind and body are interconnected, so too does the environment affect our overall health. We all have psychological reactions to colors and diversity, as well as purely physiological reactions to air quality, smells, and sounds. Unfortunately, once we become accustomed to certain surroundings, the registering of these sense stimuli seems to get bypassed through familiarity, even though their counterproductive effects can still be prominent. The first stage of creating a healthy environment is awareness. As with other components of HELP, before we can alter the factors contributing to a lack of well-being, we must first become aware of what they are.

REFLECTING ON OUR ENVIRONMENTS

Begin by reflecting on where the bulk of your time is being spent during your typical day. This may include both workplace and home, or specific rooms in these areas where you mainly spend your time. Go to these places and take time just to be with your breathing for a moment. Take a deep full breath and follow this with a relaxed prolonged exhalation. Repeat this several times with your eyes gently closed. Then open your eyes and identify the sense stimuli coming into the body as you look around the room. Become aware of smells, air quality and freshness, colors, sounds, textures, temperature, light, and shapes, and ask yourself whether the environment:

- Makes you and others who enter it feel welcome

- Gives you a sense of balance

- Promotes well-being and comfort

- Gives you a sense of connection with nature and the world around you

- Compromises your physical health in any way

- Promotes positive and meaningful interactions

- Encourages relaxation and renewal

- Reminds you of the things that are most important to you

- Promotes a degree of stimulation and creativity

- Contains elements of inspiration and beauty

- Allows for change and flexibility

The answers to all of these questions will allow you to tune into the concept of a quality environment. Look around, carefully walking into and out of the rooms. Be honest with yourself. Encourage others who visit or use these areas to go over these questions and give you feedback. Jot down these responses and ideas in your journal. Remember that as you change, as the seasons change, as the world changes around you, your environment can change also. This exercise can be repeated regularly to allow you to enhance your environment as your awareness grows.

The next step is to attune to your specific tastes and inclinations. Sit down in a comfortable and quiet space, close your eyes, and ask yourself: if you could incorporate anything at all into your environment, what would it look like? Try to be in tune with your own spirit of harmony and balance, and let go of what is fashionable or things that other people may expect. At this stage open your eyes, take out your journal and allow yourself to sketch these objects as they appear in the mind's eye. Be as specific as possible when it comes to the details. This will help to guide you when you compare your actual living and working spaces with what your inner promptings suggest.

CREATING A QUALITY ENVIRONMENT

If you have thoughtfully considered the previous exercises and questions, you are well on the way to creating a quality environment that will improve your overall health. By identifying factors that are conducive to a quality environment, as well as those that are impediments to it, you have made an immediate place to begin. Now try as much as possible to incorporate your ideal environment into your surroundings. You may add objects that are symbolic of this ideal environment—whether they be furniture, works of art, or photographs—or natural items such as flowers, plants, stones, or seashells that will allow you to connect with the outdoors even when you must be inside. Take time to create that special environment right from the start. Our tendency is not to bother addressing this issue once we have become accustomed to our present environment. Evaluate your environment on a regular basis, allowing your creative nature to flow forth with improvements and variety.

Remember the importance of the following factors, as it is estimated that most people spend 90 percent of their time indoors.

Light
Once you have become aware of your specific inclinations and tastes, devote attention to some of the primary keys for creating a quality

environment. Perhaps the most important is light. The results of numerous studies have emphasized the impact of light and color on our health. Some have even gone as far as saying that light is the second most important environmental input in controlling the functions of the body, surpassed only by food.

Wherever possible, try to reduce your dependence on artificial light and increase the flow of natural light. Evaluate how much natural light is presently flowing into the environment in which you spend the most time during daylight hours. Is there any way to increase this natural light through rearranging or redesigning the area?

Color

Color is directly associated with light. Choose colors that are agreeable to you. Learn about the properties of different colors; for example, red is stimulating, exciting, and warm, while blue tends to be relaxing, gentle, and calming. Choose colors to complement the activity that will be taking place in the specific area. Have some contrasting colors to provide a sense of variety and diversity, as it is important that colors balance one another.

Sound

Attune to sounds and noise, and try whenever possible to reduce those that are not conducive to health, such as traffic, machinery, appliances, and television. At the same time, try to be sensitive to sounds that will promote well-being, including nature sounds of birds, gentle wind chimes, and pleasant music. Take a moment to close your eyes and filter through all the sounds that come into your awareness. Identify sounds which promote ease, and those which encourage stress and anxiety.

Look at options to insulate or rearrange your environment to reduce noise, and at the same time enhance those sounds which you find healing and pleasant. If you are far from the healing sounds of the countryside, you may find audio tapes of nature sounds soothing.

Air

Next, become aware of the air flow in your environment. Air is a critical element in our overall health and well-being. Never assume that your interior environment has been designed with optimal air quality in mind. Whenever possible check into the following areas to ensure air quality:

- Look for ways to improve ventilation.

- Organize the cleaning and inspection of all air filters.

- Investigate building and insulation materials that could cause allergic reactions.

- Make sure you are able to adjust air temperature and humidity.

- Eliminate the possibility of leaks (e.g. gas) contaminating the air.

- Look for alternatives to harmful chemical cleaners for housekeeping.

- Cut down on dust particles through cleaning and leaving shoes outside.

While a great deal of attention has been focused on reducing air pollution outside it is even more critical to be aware of internal air quality.

Nature

As so much time is spent in buildings and cars, it is easy to lose the healing benefits of nature. Remember the importance of plants and items from nature to help you to:

- Attune to other living things

- Break down barriers between outdoor and indoor living

- Improve air quality and temperature

- Relax with natural colors and patterns

- Remember peaceful times outside

- Enjoy the wonder and diversity of planet Earth

This is not to mention the healing effects of looking after plants and watching them grow through your care and nurturing. By bringing nature into your indoor environment, you will be reminded of the balance and rhythm that nature represents.

People

Remember that the environment is also a product of the company you keep. The influence of the moods, attitudes, and habits of the people with whom you associate is a very significant part of environmental awareness. While it is sometimes neither desirable nor possible to surround yourself only with people who will bring out the best in you, you should be aware of the influence they have.

Seek out environments that will bring you in contact with people who can help reinforce your desire for health enhancement. Balance your social environments in order to be able to meet your goals. Choose environments that will allow you to make new friends with whom you can share your approach to life. If you are trying to let go of unhealthy habits, remember the power of being in environments where you can be with people who will assist you in this process.

When you find yourself in a difficult physical environment, try to create a pleasant atmosphere with others who are in it to help transform your thoughts and feelings. Through sharing friendship, compassion, joy, humor, and laughter, even the most difficult environments can be transformed.

SIMPLE TIPS FOR FINE-TUNING THE WORKPLACE

By allowing yourself the time and space to evaluate and change your environment, you will find that your productivity increases, your sense of peace and comfort, and your overall health and well-being improve. When looking at your workplace, identify factors that may be detrimental to your health and remedy them as much as possible. The areas mentioned previously regarding light, colors, sounds, air quality, and nature are as important in your workplace as anywhere else—or perhaps more important—although not so easily adjusted. Take time to look at your workplace from this perspective. Improve what you can in the area by applying the questions at the start of this chapter.

Be aware that modern society has affected the routine of our daily lives. Modern technology finds us sitting down a great deal more, working with machines, computers, and generally being physically inactive. Adjust for these factors by fine-tuning your work environment and making it a quality one. Special furniture and keyboards, as well as professional advice on workplace design, are available in the growing field of ergonomics. Take the time to examine your workplace with an eye toward health enhancement.

Sitting

Do you spend a great deal of time sitting? Is your chair conducive to good posture, given its height, design, and closeness to your desk? Things to look for in a good chair include:

- A support at the small of your back that can be adjusted

- A mechanism for adjusting it up and down, a tilting mechanism, and an adjustable backrest

- A wide seat

- A stable pedestal

- An appropriate height so that it fits under your desk or table and you are able to maintain good posture

If you spend a great deal of time driving, adjust your seat in a way that promotes circulation and good posture, in addition to providing comfort. The knees can be bent slightly, and a small lumbar pillow for your lower back may be helpful. Always make sure to remove things from back pockets, such as your wallet, which may not be uncomfortable, but may cause a misalignment with prolonged sitting.

Eye Stretching

Remember the importance of stretching the eyes as well as the other parts of the body. Eyestrain is a significant problem associated with our modern lifestyle. Computer screens combined with poor lighting and seating pose a formidable threat in our indoor environments.

Some simple tips to reduce eyestrain are to:

- Take frequent breaks if working in front of a screen
- Focus the eyes on objects at varying distances
- Gaze at different colors to soothe and refresh the eyes
- Remember to blink the eyes regularly
- Make sure you have good lighting

In addition, take time to do some eye exercises daily to strengthen the eye muscles and tone the optic nerves. These can include vertical, horizontal and full circular movements.

E X E R C I S E

Vertical movements:

- *Close the eyes.*
- *Slowly open the eyes, look up toward the ceiling, then lower the eyes slowly to look at the floor.*
- *Continue slow and steady up and down movements without straining or moving the head.*
- *Complete 10 rounds.*
- *Close and relax the eyes.*

Horizontal movements:

- *Close the eyes.*
- *Slowly open and move the eyes straight across the center of the vision from far right to far left.*
- *Keep the head still.*
- *Look to the periphery of the vision, repeating 10 times.*
- *Close and relax the eyes.*

Full circular movements:

- *Close the eyes.*
- *Slowly open the eyes and look up to the ceiling.*
- *Move the eyes clockwise in a full circle, passing slowly through all points.*
- *Slow the movements if the eyes jump.*

- *Speed up the movements if they are easy.*
- *Continue 10 times in one direction, then 10 times in the reverse direction.*
- *Close and relax the eyes.*

Conclude with an eye massage:

- *Close and relax the eyes.*
- *Rub the palms of the hands briskly together until they are warm.*
- *Cup the palms over the eyes.*
- *Allow the eyes to be soothed by the warmth and darkness.*
- *Lower the fingertips and gently stroke across the eyelids out toward the temples.*
- *Gently open the eyes when ready.*

There are many excellent stretches for the rest of the body which can be done in confined spaces. Some of these can be taken from the warm-up section in Chapter 2. Other stretches can be taken from the hatha yoga stretching postures illustrated in Chapter 3. Many can be done in your own office chair. Ensure that you are taking the time to stretch the body fully, and place reminders in your environment to do this, along with your positive affirmations. There are a range of books on stretching, and even ones specifically for the office, listed in the Further Reading section. Choose stretches that will allow you to improve your environmental comfort and health, while meeting your space and workplace constraints.

WEEKLY SCHEDULE

It may not be fully possible for some of you to create quality environments at home and in the workplace if you do not have control over aspects of these spaces. It is essential therefore to schedule into your diary time when you can compensate for the things which are missing or those which you cannot change. Begin by making a list, based on the pointers mentioned on page 64, of the things in your ideal environment that it is not possible to have in your actual environment. After examining the list, choose to spend as much of your free time as possible in environments that will allow you to remedy these factors. (This may seem so obvious that it should go without saying, but given the fast tempo of life today, many people are not even aware of the daily quality of environmental inputs in their lives.) For example, if you cannot redesign your office space or home to incorporate nature, ensure that during your breaks and mealtimes you take a walk, or sit in a park or garden. During weekends and holidays, choose destinations for the balance they will bring into your life, and to compensate for the environmental limitations you are faced with at most times.

Write down in your journal the aspects of your environment that you would like to change but are unable to do anything about. Review this list whenever possible, and ask these questions periodically:

- Are there any items listed that may be partially remedied by slight adjustments in your timetable for work or job definition?

- Is relocation completely out of the question, or an option you have never seriously considered?

- Where does quality environment fit into your life, and how high a priority is it?

- How aware are you on a weekly basis of the environment inputs that you have been exposed to, and what is their influence on you?

In light of this information, is it time to re-examine your priorities and perhaps move the quality of your environment higher up on the list? If it is not possible to change your environment significantly at this stage, or your priorities, at least incorporate the ideal quality inputs that are missing into your guided imagery. Remember, your body responds to what is happening in your mind as though it were real. If physical change is impossible, the mind is an excellent place in which to begin creating a quality environment.

HELPFUL HINTS FOR A QUALITY ENVIRONMENT

- Experiment with colors and how they enhance your sense of well-being.

- Learn about ergonomic adjustments to improve workplace and home.

- Discuss the concept of quality environment with coworkers and family members.

- Look at magazines and books with interior design ideas and discover what appeals to you.

- Bring your favorite aspects of nature indoors through plants, nature sounds, photos, and paintings.

- Choose music that soothes and relaxes.

- Take stretching breaks at work with coworkers.

FURTHER READING

Birren, Faber. *Light, Color and Environment,* Van Nostrand Reinhold, New York, 1982.

Friedeberger, Julie. *Office Yoga,* Thorsons, London, 1991.

Mollison, Bill & Holmgren, D. *Permaculture One,* Corgi, Bantam, Melbourne, 1978.

——*Permaculture Two,* Tagari, Hobart, Tasmania, 1979.

Venolia, Carol. *Healing Environments,* Celestial Arts, Berkeley, CA, 1988.

Wurtman, RJ. "Biological Consideration in Lighting Environments," *Progressive Architecture,* September 1973, 79-81.

Zamm, Alfred V. *Why Your House May Endanger Your Health,* Simon & Schuster, New York, 1980.

Food AWARENESS

—

AREAS OF **HELP** IN THIS CHAPTER

Understanding food awareness

•

Reflecting on current eating habits

•

Developing a healthy diet

•

Basic dietary guidelines

•

Daily routine

UNDERSTANDING FOOD AWARENESS

O f all the components of HELP, food is the most complex issue. This is an extraordinary age of abundance of food choices for those of us living in Western society. The growing, hunting, gathering, and obtaining of food are not tasks that most people, with the exception of farmers and backyard gardeners, experience anymore. Instead our food appears on the shelves of nearby supermarkets, takeout shops, and restaurants. The variety of food displayed and accessible is astounding at times, with a stream of temptations created by clever advertising and packaging, enticing smells, and the guarantees of fast, reliable, and efficient service and quality. No wonder food is such a sensitive issue. It is no longer a means by which we sustain ourselves, but has become a wonderland of choices, many of which come from a wide variety of cultures and culinary styles. Are we eating to live, or living to eat?

Now, not only do we have an abundance of foods to choose from, but we must also learn how to make the right choices, selecting foods that will be both attractive to our taste buds (which often lead us into temptation) and conducive to physical health. This is not an easy task, and it is made all the more difficult by advertising, information, diets, advice, vested business interests, and the ethnic, cultural, and family conditioning we have experienced while growing up. If we want to target healthy foods, how far do we go when confronted by choices of organic, biodynamic, minimum pesticide, no preservatives, no additives, no artificial coloring, low cholesterol, fat-free, sugar-free, low salt, no salt, no cholesterol, low cholesterol, "natural," macrobiotic, vegan … and the list goes on?

Food awareness can be very confusing. We are confronted with complex choices and bombarded with sometimes conflicting information, while being enticed by temptation and put off by alarming health studies. We have had little education in nutrition, and what information we have received about what we "should" be eating may be biased by underlying vested business interests. While our average weight is going up, the range of diets being recommended is expanding faster than people's waistlines, and the food choices continue to multiply. Will the HELP approach add yet another twist to this never-ending road of junctions, hairpin turns, dietary traffic signs, neon lights, and dead ends?

No! HELP is about awareness of the food we put into the body and, through this awareness, making decisions that will be conducive to our health. This program will not make the decisions for you. It will provide you with information that will help you to become more aware of your food choices, and assist you in ways to monitor the effects of these choices on your well-being. Unless you take the responsibility to tune into the needs of your body and the effect that certain foods have on your health, the confusion will continue unabated. Even if you understand the principles and theories behind food choices, if you are not attuned to the effects of various foods on your body, mind, and spirit, you will be a victim of your food environment rather than a master of it.

There is no question that the food or fuel we put into the body affects us. We all know that taking coffee is one way to stimulate the system, while eating large amounts of heavy foods is one way to slow it down. Yet, because of our lack of education in the area of nutrition, our food awareness is often limited to these more obvious conclusions. We need to learn the skills to fine-tune our diet in order to satisfy our needs without harming ourselves by our choices.

For a long time health professionals have directed their energies to repairing the body, rather than explaining what to put into it. Nutrition was not believed to be an appropriate subject for most medical schools. It is only recently with the compelling evidence of the importance of food awareness that things are beginning to change. These changes will hopefully lead to more information for the general public, as well as for health-care providers.

Healing Not Harming

Making the wrong food choices can be hazardous to our health. Health practitioners are now developing dietary guidelines to respond to a series of health problems including heart disease, high blood pressure, tooth decay, liver disease, obesity, diabetes, stroke, osteoporosis, gallstones, and cancers of the colon, prostate, and breast.

But at the same time as being therapeutic, proper nutrition can be a tool of prevention. Educate yourself on both your individual body and mind, and the types of food that will allow you to strengthen your body and mind given their properties and your needs. It is a simple process if you take the time to do it. Given the wide choice of foods available to us from all over the world, nature's pharmacy is at our doorstep.

In addition to acknowledging the importance of food to the maintenance of the body, research now confirms the close interrelationship between the food we eat and our psychological disposition. Not only do the foods we eat affect our moods, but also the way we feel affects our food choices. Food is a medicine of sorts, as it can produce certain effects in the system that our mind may be looking for. Like medicine, the food we eat can create moods as a result of its effect chemically on the body and mind. When we binge on food or take in excessive sweets, there is a release of endorphins—the body's natural pain-relievers—which temporarily relieve any psychological or physical pain we might have. Certain nutrients in the foods we consume have a dramatic impact on our memory, attention span, and moods. The effect of food can be like that of a drug. Developing our awareness is the only way to break the addictive habits that we may be a victim of, given this interactive dynamic of food and mood.

REFLECTING ON CURRENT EATING HABITS

The way to begin fostering food awareness is to look closely at how and what you are eating now. It may be that, with a few slight modifications, your diet and habits are completely in line with a healthy life. Or perhaps you recognize emotional patterns that seem to trigger poor eating habits on your part, and which could be overcome through greater awareness. As with all the other components of HELP, we have to develop a sense of perspective through examining our lifestyle now.

Answer the following questions in your journal. Then indicate if you can improve in any of these areas, and how you might go about doing so.

Balance

- Are you aware of balancing the foods that you eat over the course of a day, a week, a month?

- Can you sometimes not remember the last time you had fresh fruit or a salad?

- Do you actively plan your meals to ensure that you are getting a good variety of foods on a regular basis?

- Is your food balancing significantly influenced by your environment, or do you try your best to find balance wherever you are?

- Are you aware of what a balanced diet looks like?

As with every part of life, balance and moderation are the key. As highlighted throughout this guide, HELP is not a program of extremes but is always trying to maintain the integrity and harmony of body, mind, and spirit.

First, keep track of your diet over a period of time in your journal. Then evaluate it, listing percentages of the categories of foods: grains, fresh fruit, fresh vegetables, animal products (if not a vegetarian), and the occasional indulgence. Aim to have a diet which emphasizes grains, fruit and vegetables, and minimizes animal products and indulgences. Like all other aspects of HELP, food awareness must be fun and enjoyable if you are going to stick with it.

Style of Eating

Style of eating is particularly important. We can be eating the most nutritional food, but if we are rushing while eating and not chewing properly, it becomes difficult for the body to digest. Overloading the stomach when feeling anxious about upcoming events, and anticipating more to come when we have not even finished what is on our plate, results in poor digestion and the release of detrimental neurochemicals. Eat while you eat, work while you work, play while you play, and sleep while you sleep. When you mix these up, you get mixed up, and so does your body and health. It is all quite simple. Style and balance go together.

Take a moment to answer the following questions in your journal:

- Do you take your time when you eat to chew your food as much as possible?

- Are you aware of the subtle tastes?

- Do you take time to relax and let go of whatever is on your mind before eating?

- Are you aware of eating out of need rather than greed?

- Do you feel appreciative and thankful for the food that is available?

- Are you anticipating the food to come, or more of it, while still eating?

Types of Food

Given the abundance of food choices, it is often tricky to know exactly what types of food we are eating. So many different ingredients and techniques are used to make and prepare food these days for a host of reasons (cost, health, availability, mass production, appearance) that we can no longer assume what we are eating is what we think we are eating.

The food looks great, but where was it before it wound up on your plate: frozen, in a packet, in the garden? What has happened to it since that time: fried, microwaved, baked, just sliced? The answers to these questions may give you some information on its freshness, vitality, and nutritional value. If you are trying to reduce the fat content in your diet to the Heart Foundation-recommended level of below 30 percent of daily intake of calories, these factors will be helpful to know.

If you seem to develop wind after a meal, it might not be the beans, but perhaps how they were prepared, what you ate them with, how much you ate, and whatever may have still been undigested in your stomach that they were competing against. Food combinations and the quantity of food you consume may be relevant factors when examining how specific foods affect you, as much as the particular foods themselves.

Be aware of your foods now, before your body and mind force you to become aware.

- Are you aware of what is in the food you are eating?
- Are you aware of the fat content of the food?
- Do you know anything about where the food has come from or how it has been prepared?
- Is the food you are eating fresh, processed, or frozen?
- Are you aware of food combining?
- How has this type of food affected you in the past, if at all?

DEVELOPING A HEALTHY DIET

The best diet is the one that is enjoyable to you, allows you to feel good both mentally and physically, leaves you with plenty of energy, is not an ordeal to prepare, and does not harm the planet, which we all depend on for our survival. Try not to be dogmatic or evangelical in your approach; this could cause you to push your diet onto someone who is not ready, or who needs things you may not be aware of. Keep track of the foods that work for you and eliminate the ones that do not. You can share the process with others, but do not get attached to the idea that your results are for everyone.

How can you tell what is a good diet? There are some basic guidelines that just about everyone agrees upon; beyond that it is a matter of experimenting. Assume the challenging role of a detective. While simplifying your diet and testing different foods, keep good notes on your levels of energy, health, and ease of digestion and elimination. Increase your sensitivity by practicing the other components of HELP: yoga postures, breathing exercises, meditation, relaxation, mind/body awareness, group support, and so forth. Eliminate certain foods one at a time for five days and see if there is any reaction upon reintroducing them. Increase foods that help the body eliminate such as fiber-rich grains, fruit, and vegetables, then slowly introduce other foods that you would like to add and note their effect. If you have a bad reaction to a food, try it once or twice more just to verify it. Before eliminating it from your diet, check that you are combining your food properly. Adjust the times when you eat, trying to eat several smaller meals during the day to avoid eating a heavy meal before sleeping, and observe the effect.

BASIC DIETARY GUIDELINES

- Increase fruit, vegetables, and grains in your diet, thus increasing fiber consumption.

- Keep fat below 30 percent of total calorie intake, and saturated fats below 10 percent of calorie intake—the lower the better. If you have a history of heart disease, be even stricter in this area.

- Too much protein is not beneficial and need not exceed 15 percent of total calories.

- Increase unrefined carbohydrates to more than 50 percent of total calories.

- Whenever possible, consume fresh foods.

- Decrease significantly foods that have additives, or are preserved or refined (e.g. salt and sugar).

- Significantly reduce caffeine, alcohol, and chocolate.

- If you have a choice, choose certified organic or biodynamic produce.

- Be aware of your energy expenditure (e.g. is your work sedentary or physically active?) and keep food intake levels in balance. Do not overeat.

- Avoid crash or fad diets. Make dietary adjustments gradually, and increase physical exercise to burn off more calories if weight loss is desired.

- Drinking fluids, from six to eight glasses of water a day (filtered if possible), will help flush the kidneys, and reduce thirst that may be masked as hunger.

- Encourage diversity in your fruit, vegetables, juices, nuts, grains, and seeds to fulfill vitamin and mineral needs.

- Enjoy your food while eating it, no matter what it is. Your attitude toward it is very important for your own physical, mental, emotional, and spiritual well-being. Do not feel guilty about the occasional indulgence. Food should be fun!

If you have a specific ailment, you should seek out specialized diets. The above guidelines reflect more of what is traditionally known as a maintenance diet for good health.

DAILY ROUTINE

Making the changes in daily patterns of behavior that will allow you to break the habits of many years is not easy, but it is possible through dedication and discipline. Rather than trying to meet all the above guidelines, set goals which target the areas that you need to work on the most. Be aware of other parts of your life that may conflict with these goals (e.g. social commitments, partner, and so on), and seek a happy compromise. Begin with goals that are realistic, such as "I will try to reduce my current consumption of fat to a level less than 30 percent of total calorie intake over the next two months," (if that is realistic for you), rather than "I will never have any foods that contain saturated fat" (if you suspect that is unlikely). Try also to be specific, with targets that are measurable and attainable within a given time context.

Create a detailed picture of the type of diet you are striving for and use it as a model. Write it down and visualize it as clearly as possible in the mind's eye whenever sitting down to eat. Take a moment before eating to ask yourself whether you are living this goal. The more specific the diet is, the easier this will be.

Be clear as to what the achievement of this diet means to you in terms of your own emotions, physical well-being, mental peace, or other desires you might have. Make a commitment to it by knowing how important it is to you, and what you are willing to do to achieve it.

Have a plan as to how you will be able to implement this diet, taking into consideration how the diet may be challenged through eating in restaurants and at friends' homes, eating takeout, your partner's desires, your job functions, workplace limitations, and so forth.

Be flexible: if for some reason you are challenged in a way that you least expect, try to adapt and adjust, remembering to enjoy the journey of food awareness. If you fail at first, do not get discouraged but rather be a bit more realistic in your plan and forgive yourself. The next day, start afresh with full commitment.

When you are successful, take some time out (perhaps at the end of the day) to pat yourself on the back, boosting both your motivation and spirits. It is important to enjoy your accomplishments.

Enlist the support of family, friends, and others, by telling them of your goals and asking them to assist you if possible. At least they will understand why you have chosen to be more aware of food without seeking to convert them. Seek out like-minded people and books, or other sources of information such as cooking classes or nutritionists, to answer questions that come up, and reinforce your commitment.

Above all, have a sense of humor, remembering the journey is to be enjoyed. Give yourself a break, and do not be in too great a hurry to change overnight. It is far better to begin slowly and adhere fully to your plan than to set unrealistic goals and meet them once every four days.

Through food awareness, combined with the other HELP components, you will be able to maintain the weight that is right for you. You will have an easeful body that takes you where you want to go, and a tranquil mind allowing you to enjoy the wonders of life.

HELPFUL HINTS FOR FOOD AWARENESS

- Eat according to your level of hunger, and stop before you are absolutely full.

- Select the amount of food according to your own daily energy needs.

- Try to eat at regular set times to develop a routine of digestion.

- Try not to eat late at night, leaving a minimum of 2 hours before sleeping.

- Be aware of chewing your food as much as possible and the taste of each bite.

- Eat with a calm mind.

- Leave newspapers, books, and phone calls aside and EAT WHILE YOU EAT.

- Try to eat in a quality environment that is conducive to enjoying your food.

- Choose restaurants that you know will have healthy food selections.

- Accept yourself no matter what you have eaten, letting go of guilt.

FURTHER READING

Ballentine, Rudolph. *Diet and Nutrition,* Himalayan International Institute of Yoga Science, Honesdale, PA, 1978.

Department of Health and Human Services (US), Public Health Service. *The Surgeon-General's Report on Nutrition and Health,* Government Printing Office, Washington, DC, 1988.

Ornish, Dean. *Eat More Weigh Less,* HarperCollins, New York, 1993.

Robbins, J. *Diet for a New America,* EarthSave, Felton, Stillpoint Publishing, Walpole, New Hampshire, 1987.

Wurtman, RJ. "Behavioural Effects of Nutrients," *Lancet,* 1(8334), 1145–1147.

The Mind/Body CONNECTION

AREAS OF **HELP** IN THIS CHAPTER

Understanding the mind/body connection

•

Mind/body reflection

•

Activating mind/body harmony

•

The humor prescription

•

Weekly schedule

UNDERSTANDING THE MIND/BODY CONNECTION

One of the most exciting areas of health research in recent years has been the discovery of the connection between the mind and the physical body through neurotransmitters. Major changes in health care are now taking place as a result of greater understanding of how the mind/body dynamic works. From runner's high and endorphins, to biofeedback and imagery, the language of the mind/body connection is making its way into daily life.

We are all aware of the fact that our thoughts and feelings have a direct impact on body functions, such as when a feeling of embarrassment from someone's remark causes our face to blush. We hear a strange sound when we are alone at night in the house. Perhaps someone is threatening our security. Our breathing becomes fast and shallow. We experience nervous tension in the body, sweaty palms, a pounding heart, and a general feeling of unease. When we discover it is just a strong breeze causing a tree branch to rub against the house—when the mental thought of threat is released—all our symptoms disappear.

The thoughts that we have each moment send a chemical response from the brain via the nervous system to affect all parts of the body, including the functioning of our immune system.

Hence the terms *psycho*—the mind, *neuro*—the nervous system of communication linkages in the body, and *immunology*—the ability of the body to stay healthy through warding off dis-ease. Psychoneuroimmunology (PNI) allows us to see the effects of negative thoughts, ideas, and emotions, in terms of how they suppress the immune function, and also to learn about the chemicals that can be released to help strengthen the immune system.

As a result of these findings, we can actually begin to tap into the internal pharmacy of the body. We can begin to learn how to produce chemical releases through our thoughts, emotions, and actions that will help us maintain or rehabilitate the physical body.

This is not to imply in any way that the HELP approach precludes consulting with your health professional or to suggest that you forego recommended treatments prescribed by them in favor of positive thinking. The HELP approach is complementary, and when research is referred to in this context it is always with this complementary approach in mind; rather than one approach being an "alternative" to the other. It may be possible to reduce prescriptions or avoid surgery, but always make these decisions in consultation with your health professional.

While researchers are still examining the communication network between mind and body, the basic conclusions thus far indicate there is a continuous dialogue between the nervous, immune, and endocrine systems, whereby emotions influence immunity—uplifting emotions bolster it and negative emotions depress it. These systems release and receive messenger molecules called neuropeptides in response to anything other than normal functions that are triggered in the body such as anxiety, invading bacteria, and extreme temperature change. Neuropeptides carry a variety of messages dependent on their origins and their goal. Peptides can direct immune system cells, which can cause you to feel pain, raise or lower the body temperature, and influence emotional feelings of joy or depression.

While neuroscientists are busy exploring the nature of this communication system and the full range of neurotransmitters, other health professionals have been developing a range of studies to determine how our state of mind—particularly levels of stress, relaxation, hope, fear, laughter, isolation, intimacy, and service—may affect the body on a physiological level.

One of the better known studies conducted over 20 years ago by Dr Herbert Benson of the Harvard Medical School demonstrated that people who practiced what he calls the relaxation response, a state of profound rest produced through mental concentration, could reduce heart rate, lower blood pressure, reduce oxygen consumption, and lower the breathing rate. In addition, through this state of concentration the brain waves shifted from the alert beta-rhythm to the relaxed alpha-rhythm. Other changes included a decrease in blood flow to the muscles and an increase in blood to the skin and brain, resulting in a feeling of warmth and rested mental alertness.

Dr Benson's study is one of literally thousands that have been and are now being done in order to assist people and medical science learn more about who gets sick, and how our beliefs, moods, thoughts, lifestyle, and environment affect our health. In addition to these factors, we must always remember that our genetic constitution and behavior are also determinants of health. While heredity is beyond our personal control, the many other factors can be worked with, and they form the basis of the HELP approach.

Dr George Solomon of the University of California, Los Angeles, often called the "father of psychoneuroimmunology," began investigating the mind/body interaction 30 years ago, before it had become an accepted discipline. He has applied his research in the field of psychiatry, examining how personality may affect the capacity of the body's immune system to fend off illnesses including cancer, AIDS, rheumatoid arthritis, viral infections, and lupus.

The profile of an immunologically healthy person, according to Dr Solomon includes:

- Being in touch with their bodily and psychological needs

- Being able to meet those needs by assertive action

- Possessing coping skills, including a sense of control, that enables them to ward off depression

- Having the ability to express emotions, including anger and sadness

- Being willing to ask for and accept support from loved ones

- Having a sense of meaning and purpose in their daily activities, including work and relationships

- Having a capacity for pleasure and play

Health researchers are finding that people who develop these skills are far more likely to survive AIDS, cancer, and other diseases. Scientists are now able to document changes in the various white blood cells involved in this process. Other findings have indicated the positive effects of diet, physical exercise, environment, and stress-management techniques on the mind/body equation.

As technology continues to advance, and as neuroscientists keep probing, thousands of messengers will be uncovered. However, we do not have to wait for those discoveries to begin to derive the benefits from these findings. The process can start now with the 12 components of HELP. By having an integrated, healthy lifestyle we can develop a strong immune function and a joyful outlook on life.

MIND/BODY REFLECTION

The success of all HELP components will be determined by our outlook on life. An analogy that we are all familiar with is the planting of a seed. No matter what the potential of the seed, unless the soil is appropriate, the climate suitable, and care is taken to look after it, the plant will not grow properly or remain healthy. The HELP approach is like a wonderful seed that can grow and unleash powerful energy and vibrant health in your life. Take the time to reflect on your approach to life. This is the existing soil. Enrich the soil by making a commitment to the points above. Examine the environment you work and live in. This is the climate. Bring sunshine and joy into it to promote growth. Then take care and look after the HELP seed with attention, and experience mind/body harmony.

Take some time for reflection, open your journal and answer the questions below:

- When was the last time you had a good laugh at yourself and the situations you find yourself in?
- Are you holding any grudges, animosities, and wounds? If so, what are they?
- Do you take time out to reflect back on difficult times in your life?
- Were there any positive repercussions of these adversities?
- Can you see adversity as an impetus for growth in your life?
- What are you ultimately responsible for that no one else has a role in? List your answers.
- Now ask yourself: how do the items on this list differ from the things that you take upon yourself that you have little control over?

- Have you learned to accept those things over which you have little or no control?

- Do you tackle challenges with a spirit of curiosity and wonder?

This reflection serves as a starting point for the journey of enhancing the quality of your life. As you continue with the components of HELP, become aware of the interactive nature of the program. How your thoughts influence your physical well-being, as well as how looking after your body through food awareness, exercise, and yoga uplifts your mental health. Take time out to answer these questions again as you progress with HELP.

ACTIVATING MIND/BODY HARMONY

Each component of the HELP lifestyle program is designed to enhance the mind/body connection, allowing you to acquire skills and empower yourself. The following points serve as a foundation for bringing greater harmony and flow through all 12 components of HELP:

- Make a point to share a laugh and express your sense of humor.

- Take time to tune into your needs and nourish and love yourself.

- Let go of wounds, and take steps to heal relationships.

- Realize your need for intimacy, and develop honest, fun, and loving relationships.

- Look at the positive and uplifting side when confronted with the challenges of life.

- Nurture a childlike sense of curiosity and wonder about the world.

- Accept yourself and those around you, and see life as a growth experience.

- Forgive others and yourself, as you let go of negative emotions of resentment and envy.

- Develop positive images and goals to guide you in your endeavors.

- Allow yourself to experience joy, delight, and peace, while sharing them with others.

- Take a step back and witness the events of the week with a sense of equanimity.

If you lack vitality, peace of mind, and physical well-being, it may be that one or more of the above are not currently a significant part of your life. To some extent, we all need HELP, to assist us to keep this perspective and develop a lifestyle program that will increase the quality of our lives.

THE HUMOR PRESCRIPTION

The most joyful and easily accessible approach to mind/body harmony is humor. While other HELP components will provide assistance with the physical, mental, social, and environmental factors associated with mind/body harmony, it is clearly the case that laughter and humor are fundamental keys to the quality of life. Many research studies have documented what we already know: *it feels great to laugh*. For those still needing proof, the following physiological responses are all associated with laughter:

- Increase in muscle relaxation and resulting decrease in anxiety

- Release of endorphins and catecholamines, the body's natural chemicals for boosting energy and euphoric feelings

- Increased oxygenation of the blood

- Initial increase in heart rate, then arteries relax and heart rate and blood pressure lower

- Stimulation of immune response through reduced cortisol secretion

If laughter had been recently discovered and was sold by pharmacists, it would be prescribed as an antidote for a wide variety of ailments. Yet humor's power as a remedy for body and mind has failed to make its way into mainstream medicine. Laughter provides a healing environment. From a social and psychological perspective, there are few antidotes more effective than laughter. It helps to release stress, promotes camaraderie, and is a key indicator of mental health. When we can no longer laugh at ourselves, depression and alienation are not far behind.

A WEEKLY SCHEDULE

To increase the laughter and humor in your life is easy. Once we know how important it is to our health, make a commitment to joy as your medium. Know that it will not only enhance your health but all you come in contact with. When is the last time you avoided being with someone who made you laugh and feel good about life? Who is the life of the party? He who laughs last is a fool for waiting so long.

Use humorous affirmations to keep you attuned to joy. Remember funny phrases, incidents, or stories and recall them during the day. Remind yourself that you are funny and life can be playful. It may be as simple as wearing brightly colored socks or mismatching them as a reminder not to get too serious during the day. Your birthright is joy and peace. Know that this life could end at any moment, and how nice it would be to go out with a smile on your face, a humorous thought, a skip in your step, or just having brought joy into someone's life.

Reframe your perspective to find humor in the challenges that you face. I remember a time when my grandfather was dying of lung cancer and staying in our home. He had only a few weeks to live and was sleeping outside on a lounge chair being warmed by the summer sun. We were inside attending to lunch preparations when Grandpa came in with a fresh bird dropping on the top of his bald head. We felt like crying on seeing him there. What else could happen to this poor man in the few remaining days of his life. He immediately shared his gift of life that had carried him through years of challenge. In a weak and raspy voice he announced it was a joyous sign of good fortune, as he had been sleeping with his mouth wide open, and if it hadn't been for God's grace and good luck it might have landed on his tongue. We all burst out laughing. He had reframed the situation for all of us.

HELPFUL HINTS FOR MIND/BODY JOY

Use the following tools to stimulate your imagination, sense of play, wonderment, curiosity, and joy! These can be particularly good reminders when life and the news around you seem to carry little to laugh about. Add your favorite fun ideas to the following suggestions:

• Have cartoon and joke books always out on tables or nearby.

• Wear a red nose, silly clothes, face paint, funny glasses, a silly hat.

• Listen to or create enjoyable music.

• Read a storybook or fairy tale to allow the imagination to flow.

• Laugh aloud in the most unlikely places regularly.

• Sing fun songs.

• Develop wonderful unexpected sounds and voices that delight.

• Buy magic and fun shop props.

• Make a list of people and situations that have ushered in joyful feelings.

• Plan comedy nights with family, friends, or coworkers.

• Organize humorous skits and drama get-togethers.

• Remember to play—play games, play on the beach, play with words, play with children.

• Learn to juggle.

• View comedy shows or funny movies; listen to comedy recordings.

• Enjoy the sunset or sunrise with someone.

• Practice making funny faces in a mirror and try them out in public.

• Call an old friend and recall a funny incident you shared together.

FURTHER READING

Adams, Patch with Mylander, Maureen. *Gesundheit!*, Healing Arts Press, Rochester, Vermont, 1993.

Benson, Herbert. *The Mind/Body Effect*, Simon & Schuster, New York, 1979.

Borysenko, J. *Minding the Body, Mending the Mind*, Bantam Books, New York, 1988.

Cousins, Norman. *Head First*, Dutton, New York, 1989.

Chernin, Dennis, MD & Manteuffel, Gregory, MD. *Health: A Holistic Approach*, Quest, London, 1984.

Ekman, P, Levenson, RW & Friesen, WV. "Autonomic Nervous System Activity Distinguishes among Emotions," *Science*, 221 (4616) 1983, 1208-10.

Goleman, Daniel & Gurin, Joel (eds). *Mind Body Medicine*, Consumer Reports Books, New York, 1993.

Jaffe, Dennis T. *Healing from Within: Psychological Techniques to Help the Mind and Body*, Fireside/Simon & Schuster, New York, 1986.

Justice, Blair. *Who Gets Sick: How Beliefs, Moods, and Thoughts Affect Your Health*, Jeremy P Tarcher, Los Angeles, 1987.

Moody, Raymond Jr. *Laugh After Laugh: The Healing Power of Humor*, Headwaters Press, Jacksonville, FL, 1978.

Moyers, Bill. *Healing and the Mind*, Doubleday, New York, 1993.

Solomon, George. "The Emerging Field of Psychoneuroimmunology with a Special Note on AIDS," *Advances*, 2 (1), 1985.

——Interview in *Natural Health*, January/February 1992, 52-59.

Siegel, Bernie S. *Love, Medicine and Miracles*, Harper & Row, New York, 1986.

——*Peace, Love and Healing*, Rider, Sydney, 1990.

Breath of LIFE

—

AREAS OF **HELP** IN THIS CHAPTER

Understanding the power of breath

•

The science of breathing

•

Reflecting on breath awareness

•

Guidelines for breathing practices

•

Abdominal breathing

•

Deep three-part breathing

•

Rapid diaphragmatic breathing

•

Alternate nostril breathing

•

Suggested daily practice

UNDERSTANDING THE POWER OF BREATH

B reath has a significant effect on the mind and body. It may seem difficult to understand at first that such a simple thing as breathing can have a major impact on our health. We are all familiar with how our breath changes according to what we are doing and thinking. If the breath is affected by both body and mind, is it not possible that by changing the patterns of the breathing we can then reverse this process and use breathing as a vehicle to affect both body and mind? This chapter is about your breathing, its importance to health, and techniques to harness the power of the breath. The benefits range from helping to balance your nervous system and enhancing your energy levels, to calming your mind.

In the HELP program, breath is seen as a crucial connection between your body and mind. When we are angry and upset our breathing tends to be very rapid and shallow, illustrating the link with our thoughts and emotions. A sob of grief, a yawn of tiredness or boredom, a sigh of resignation are just a few of the other signals of this connection with the mind. Of course, not only does the mind affect the breath but changes in our bodies also affect our breath. For example, when we walk briskly or jog up a hill, the exercise increases our oxygen requirements and we therefore breathe faster and deeper to bring more oxygen or energy into the body to cope with this exertion.

THE SCIENCE OF BREATHING

There is a whole science of breath based on yoga breathing practices called *pranayama*. This science guides us in becoming aware of the connections between the breath and the rest of our functions. It also shows us how to alter our breathing patterns to directly promote positive changes in our body and mind. Breath is no longer just a result of mental or physical changes but becomes a tool to affect them. According to these teachings, *prana* is energy or the vital force, and the breath is the vehicle for prana in and out of the body. *Yama* means control, and so these pranayama practices allow us to gain control of this energy, and to be able to use it to improve our health.

We can survive for many days without food and water, but without breathing we would cease to exist in this physical body in just a few minutes. In normal breathing, we use only the upper portions of the lungs. The breath tends to be shallow. By altering this breathing pattern and using full abdominal breaths, we can move 8 to 10 times the volume of air moved by our shallow normal breaths. While breathing is an autonomic bodily function that carries on essentially on its own, we do have the capacity to change our pattern of breathing consciously through awareness and practice, and thus improve the quality of our lives.

If the breath is so crucial to our overall health, why are most of us not breathing more deeply now, and how did shallow breathing come about? First, despite the physiological evidence regarding the importance and actual dynamics of breathing, most of us have never been informed about the power of the breath and its impact on mind and body by our health practitioners or teachers. When we breathe from our chest only, the breath is usually irregular and rapid, which triggers stressful feelings and occasionally the fight-or-flight response in the mind and body. Also, on an anatomical basis, the lower portion of the lungs have the greatest amount of blood flow, and with shallow chest breathing there is very little oxygen getting to this crucial part of the lungs. By altering this pattern and deepening the breath—instead of an anxiety reaction in the body and a limited amount of oxygen being absorbed into the bloodstream—we can produce a sense of calm, a greater alertness of mind and a healthier body through a greater flow of oxygen.

In addition to the lack of education about the importance of deep breathing, there are several other factors that account for shallow breathing. Accumulated anxiety and emotional trauma cause our abdomens to become tight and this stops us from taking deep inhalations. Another factor is our lifestyles. Due to advances in technology, we are far more sedentary than ever before and, without exercise, our breathing becomes shallow. Finally, many people have been encouraged in their early years to create a "desirable" posture, by sucking in their belly and puffing out their chest. This practice undermines proper breathing, as it constricts the abdominal muscles and makes it impossible to take in full deep inhalations. The good news is that we can develop control of our breathing. Through greater awareness and the practices that follow in this chapter, all of these obstacles can be removed.

REFLECTING ON BREATH AWARENESS

The first step is to reflect on how you are breathing right now. This technique will allow you to establish a base point from which you can make improvements and learn to breathe properly. Record observations of your breathing in your journal to compare with later periods. Include:

- Rhythm
- Depth
- Sound
- Body movements

EXERCISE

Sitting with your spine straight, head, neck and trunk in alignment, place your right hand on your chest and your left hand on your abdomen. Without trying to change the flow of breath from its natural rhythm, just observe the movement of the hands. If your right hand rises more than your left hand, then you are breathing from your chest. If your left hand rises more than your right, then you are breathing from your abdominal area. Again, just observe the next few breaths and take note of how you are breathing now. Are you breathing through your nose or your mouth? Is your breath flowing and smooth? Notice the sound of your breath. Once you have been practicing breathing techniques for a while you will be able to compare your breathing.

GUIDELINES FOR BREATHING PRACTICES

A few guiding principles are worth mentioning before introducing some of the breathing practices that will help transform both your breathing pattern and your well-being. Always try whenever possible to breathe through the nose. The nose has been designed to act as a filter for the air, as well as warming the air before it enters the lungs. Be aware of your posture, particularly your shoulders: they should be held back without being stiff. It is best to have the chest cavity as open as possible to help promote deep breathing. Try to focus the mind on the technique that you are employing. The mind will have a tendency to drift off to other areas once you have learned the specific practice. When the mind strays it may very well affect both your posture and the actual technique itself. For maximum benefit, try to keep the awareness always with the breathing technique you are practicing. The breathing techniques, while simple, must be taken seriously and practiced regularly in order to reverse patterns of breathing that have developed over a lifetime. The cautions are the following:

- If at any time you feel light-headed or dizzy, discontinue the technique and return the breath to normal until steadiness returns.

- Never do the practices to extreme. Follow the instructions and gradually build up your capacity.

- If you wish to go beyond the techniques given here, do so only under the guidance of an instructor qualified in pranayama.

- Do not underestimate the power of the breath and its ability to transform your health if done properly, or to be detrimental if instructions are not followed.

ABDOMINAL BREATHING

As most of us are breathing from our upper chest, the first technique is to learn abdominal breathing so as to allow us to deepen the breath and feel less stressed and more balanced.

EXERCISE

Begin by checking your posture, taking in a deep breath and then exhaling as much air as you possibly can as you fully contract the abdominal muscles. If you want to place one hand on the abdomen to ensure that it is pulling in fully on the exhalation, feel free to do so. This full exhalation will force out all the stale air from the lower portion of the lungs, and the resulting effect is one of a vacuum, which will pull in a nice deep inhalation with the abdomen expanding out like a balloon. Always remember, as you continue this practice over the next few minutes, that the abdomen is expanding out on the inhalation and all the abdominal muscles are contracting on the exhalation, causing the belly to flatten. If you happen to be a reverse breather and find that your natural breath involves your abdomen expanding on the exhalation and contracting on the inhalation, then you will have to practice this technique as much as possible to retrain yourself to breathe in the correct manner.

If you experience difficulty in isolating the abdominal part from the rest of your breath, just lie down on the floor on your back with your arms relaxed and slightly away from the body, and your feet shoulder width apart. Now place a small, light weight on your abdomen, such as a little sandbag, thin book, or other similar object. Concentrating on the object, just observe it rising and falling with each respiration. This will give you a physical point of reference to focus on while deepening and changing your breathing pattern. If this practice seems strange or unnatural at first, give it time and through regular sessions this abdominal breathing will become automatic.

DEEP THREE-PART BREATHING

This practice incorporates the abdominal breathing you have just learned and takes it further. It is an excellent practice for stress management as well as for improving the supply of oxygen into the body. Because you take your breathing wherever you go, this practice can be done at any time. You may find it particularly useful in breaking the anxiety cycle, by altering your reaction to external circumstances that are beyond your control. If you feel a sense of worry or anger building up in an anxious moment, just practice this technique to help calm the body and mind, and thereby change your reaction to the situation.

E X E R C I S E

Again, begin by checking your posture—head, neck, and trunk in a straight line, with the shoulders back but not stiff. Placing your right hand on your chest and your left hand on the abdomen, exhale completely through your nose. Begin inhaling by filling your abdominal area and allowing it to expand out like a balloon. During this expansion your left hand should begin to rise while the right hand is not moving.

After filling your abdominal area, keep the inhalation flowing as you allow the air to rise up and fill your lower chest. This should cause the right hand to rise and the ribcage to expand. Keep inhaling as you now let the air flow into the upper chest. As the air reaches the top of your lungs the collarbones will rise slightly. The lungs are now almost completely filled with air as a result of this three-part technique. First the abdomen, then the lower chest, and finally the upper chest.

Now exhaling, repeat the same process but in reverse from top to bottom. Begin by exhaling and releasing air from the upper chest, allowing the collarbones to fall. Then continue to exhale from the upper chest while moving down to the lower chest, feeling it beginning to contract. Conclude with the abdominal area and expel all the remaining air by contracting the abdominal muscles fully.

Continue this practice with your next inhalation: abdomen, lower chest and upper chest, and exhale in the reverse order. Practice for a few minutes to become familiar with the dynamics of deep three-part breathing.

The benefits of the deep, three-part breath are many. In addition to the stress-management application already mentioned (by transforming your shallow breaths), this technique will allow you gradually to increase your lung capacity. It will have a noticeable effect on your energy level and mental clarity as a result of greater oxygenation of the blood. It is also particularly beneficial for people suffering with chronic lung and bronchial conditions.

RAPID DIAPHRAGMATIC BREATHING

The greater awareness of the abdominal muscles gained from the previous two techniques provides a good basis for this next practice, which involves vigorous expulsion of breath using the diaphragm and abdominal muscles, followed by a relaxation of the abdominal area resulting in a slow, natural inhalation. The emphasis is placed on the exhalation, on making it rapid and forceful. The exhalation is immediately followed by a relaxed inhalation replacing the air expelled. This practice is particularly helpful if you are feeling sluggish, as it is very good for boosting energy levels.

E X E R C I S E

Check the posture as before. Inhale fully, then exhale forcefully a small quantity of air and immediately follow this with a natural inhalation. Only the abdominal muscles should be moving: they contract with the rapid forceful exhalations, then release to allow the air to flow in with each relaxed inhalation. Again, you may wish to put your hand on the abdomen to ensure that this abdominal action is taking place with each breath. Once you become accustomed to the action of the breath, begin to increase the frequency of the breathing to about two exhalations and inhalations per second. When beginning, start with between 15 and 20 forceful exhalations, followed by relaxed inhalations. On the last exhalation, expel a larger quantity of air, then take a deep three-part breath, followed by a slow relaxed exhalation.

This constitutes one round. After allowing the breath to return to normal, do two more rounds when you are ready. Again, if at any time you feel discomfort, immediately return your breath back to normal.

ALTERNATE NOSTRIL BREATHING

The alternate nostril breathing practice is one of the most beneficial and powerful of the breathing techniques. While most people are not aware of it, during the day the flow of air through your nose shifts from predominantly one nostril to the other, changing for most people at about two-hourly intervals. This technique has been designed to ensure a state of balanced breathing through each of the nostrils. Upon completing the practice, people generally feel a calming and relaxing sensation in both mind and body. It has a soothing and strengthening effect on the nervous system, increases mental alertness, and helps to cleanse and open the nasal passages.

While medical science has yet to go beyond acknowledging that this shifting of nostrils and breathing patterns does take place, there is, according to yogic texts, a direct linkage between this breathing pattern and the mind. It is generally recognized that the different hemispheres of the brain are responsible for different functions.

The right side of the brain is responsible not only for the motor functions of the left side of the body but also for orientation in space, artistic ability, and our capacity for recognizing familiar places and people. This right hemisphere possibly serves an integrating function, allowing us to respond to a situation as a whole. People who have suffered injuries to this hemisphere experience difficulties in these areas while other brain motor functions remain intact.

The left side of the brain is responsible for the right side of the body, and controls verbal skills, logical thinking, and mathematical functions. It deals with cause-and-effect relationships, and inputs in a sequential fashion.

In the yoga approach to breathing, when you are breathing predominantly through the left nostril you are activating the right side of the brain, and thus stimulating the activities associated with that hemisphere; and vice versa. When the breath flows evenly through one nostril and then the other, both hemispheres are in balance, producing a sense of calm and relaxation.

E X E R C I S E

To practice this technique, sit in a comfortable position, and once again check your posture, ensuring the head, neck and trunk are in a straight line, the spine is straight but not stiff, the shoulders are back, and the body is relaxed. Now make a gentle fist with your right hand, releasing the thumb and the last two fingers. The technique is to block off the right nostril with the thumb while breathing through the left nostril, and then alternate. Exhale fully. Now place the thumb against the right nostril and inhale through the left nostril. At the completion of the inhalation release the thumb, close off the left nostril with the ring finger and exhale through the right nostril. Next inhale through the right nostril and, at the completion of the inhalation, block the right nostril off with the thumb and exhale through the left nostril, releasing the ring finger. Continue this pattern: exhale, inhale, then switch nostrils. Change nostrils after each inhalation.

Once you feel comfortable with the dynamics of the technique, work toward making the exhalation longer than the inhalation, with it eventually being twice as long as the inhalation. The breath should be flowing smoothly and deeply throughout the technique, and you should be using a correct posture. Again, if at any time you feel like you are not getting enough air or feel light-headed or dizzy, discontinue the practice and return your breath to normal. Continue this technique for up to 2 minutes. If your arm gets tired, just bring the elbow in toward your chest. When you are ready to conclude, finish on the exhalation through the right nostril and allow the breath to return to normal, then sit quietly for a moment with your eyes gently closed.

SUGGESTED DAILY PRACTICE

To begin this program it is suggested that you allot a minimum of 5 minutes daily for the breathing practices in conjunction with your other program activities. You may start with 30 seconds of abdominal breathing, a minute and a half of deep three-part breathing, a minute of rapid diaphragmatic breathing, and conclude with 2 minutes of alternate nostril breathing. Once you feel comfortable with the practices and techniques, slowly begin to increase the time you spend doing them. Again, make the increases in time gradual, giving your body a smooth transition and working within your limits and toward realistic goals.

When wanting to extend the practice of rapid diaphragmatic breathing, begin by increasing the number of exhalations per round from 15 to 20, to 20 to 25, never exceeding increases of 5 at any stage. After each increase, wait three weeks before the next one. Always be gradual in the process and, again, if you notice any disconcerting states or difficulties, return the breathing to normal at once. The key is regular practice rather than increasing the number of rounds once a week to make up for times you have missed. Through gradual and steady increases that are sustained daily, the maximum benefit will come to you.

Alternate nostril breathing should be approached on the same basis. Slowly extend the time you do the practice, by up to 30 seconds at a time. Practice that increase daily for at least one week, and make sure you can handle it comfortably before making any further increases. Also, be aware of building up the length of the exhalation, eventually trying to make the exhalation twice as long as the inhalation. Proceed slowly when working on extending the exhalation. You should not feel like you are gasping for the next inhalation. The breath should be quiet, smooth, and steady. You may wish to count, initially inhaling to a count of 4 and exhaling to a count of 8. Gradually work the exhalation up to a count of 10. When you have been able to sustain that for at least three weeks, increase the inhalation to 6 and the exhalation to 12, as you are able to do so. Using the same formula of waiting at least three weeks to build up your capacity, and monitoring the effects, aim to breathe for 3 minutes at a count of 10 for each inhalation and a count of 20 for each exhalation, without gasping, and keeping the breath quiet and smooth.

Try to incorporate deep three-part breathing as much as possible into your awareness, using the abdominal muscles as frequently as you can when breathing throughout the day—whatever you are doing. The abdominal breathing and deep three-part breathing should be practiced as much as possible, whenever and wherever you find yourself, to help develop a whole new pattern of breathing and a wonderful range of benefits for body and mind.

Daily breathing practice with awareness will help to transform your overall health, bringing vitality, balance, and energy into your life. The breath is a wonderful tool for both body and mind. By becoming more aware of your breathing patterns, and slowly changing them, you will experience the dynamic power of the breath of life.

HELPFUL HINTS FOR BREATHING PRACTICES

- Put a reminder simply saying "bp" on your office wall, in your wallet, by your bed.

- Get together with others who may be interested in improving their health, and share these practices.

- Join a yoga class that has breathing practices as part of the class.

- Use an audiotape to help guide you through your routine.

- When out in the country or at the beach take advantage of fresh clean air with deep breathing.

- Never pass up the chance to blow up balloons, air mattresses, and beach balls.

- Exercise regularly to help develop lung capacity.

FURTHER READING

Rama, Swami, Ballantine, Rudolph & Hymes, Alan. *The Science of Breath: A Practical Guide,* Himalayan International Institute of Yoga Science, Honesdale, PA, 1979.

Satchidananda, S. *To Know Your Self,* Anchor Books, New York, 1978.

——*Integral Yoga Hatha,* Holt, Rinehart & Winston, New York, 1975.

Speads, Carola. *Ways to Better Breathing,* Healing Arts Press, Rochester Vermont, 1978.

A Peaceful
MIND

___

AREAS OF HELP IN THIS CHAPTER

Understanding meditation

•

Benefits of meditation

•

Reflecting on the nature of the mind

•

Preparing for meditation

•

Dealing with mental distractions

•

Techniques for concentrating the mind

•

Suggested daily program

UNDERSTANDING MEDITATION

We have all experienced the benefits of peaceful and meditative moments at some point in our lives, whether we were aware of them at the time or not. Perhaps when walking along the beach, completely absorbed in the moment. No thoughts of the past, no plans for the future. Making no distinctions, judgments, or comparisons in the mind, just feeling at one with our surroundings. At one with the sand, the waves, the sea breeze, the universe. Completely at peace, totally absorbed and focused in the moment. Allowing ourselves just to be.

While this may be a fleeting and random occurrence, it need not be if we choose to make meditation a part of our daily lives. The practice of meditation has been utilized for thousands of years, and it is neither complex nor associated with any particular religion or doctrine. It is available to people whatever their background or belief structure, and requires no conversion or abandonment of a present spiritual orientation. It goes by many different names, including the relaxation response, centering, transcendental meditation (TM), and the calm technique, to name a few. Meditation can enable you to experience the deep reservoir of peace within you, no matter where you are, whether at the beach or in your home. Once you become familiar with it, you can gain the benefits wherever you happen to be.

The practice of meditation is the culmination of a process which involves two preliminary steps:

1. Withdrawing awareness from the sense stimuli of sound, taste, touch, sight, and smell.

2. Concentrating the mind by using a technique to gradually focus the mental energies, allowing the mind to become one-pointed and focused beyond distraction.

Once the mind is completely still and focused, the meditation process is fully engaged and its benefits are forthcoming. The mind is no longer responding to external stimuli, and has gone beyond its erratic state of skipping from one image, thought, or idea to another. The mind becomes completely focused on the object of concentration.

BENEFITS OF MEDITATION

When in a meditative state, a sense of profound peace is experienced, and medical researchers have found correspondingly positive physiological changes to occur. These benefits include:

- Reduction in blood pressure
- Release of muscular tension in the body
- Slowing down of the heartbeat
- Reduction in the rate of respiration
- Reduction in the metabolic rate
- Increase in the slower, more relaxed "alpha" waves of the brain
- Decrease in blood lactate levels
- Reduction in oxygen consumption
- Increase in skin resistance to electrical impulse
- Decrease in gastric acid secretion

In addition to these physiological responses, people who meditate regularly report feeling a heightened awareness through focusing the mind, a greater sense of relaxation, and a breaking down of feelings of isolation. As Dr Dean Ornish has shown in his landmark research on reversing heart disease, people who feel isolated have three to five times the rate of mortality, not only from heart disease but from all causes of death, compared with those who have a greater sense of intimacy. Isolation can often lead to feelings of chronic stress and emotional pain. We can be isolated from others, from a higher force, from our bodies, from our feelings, and from our inner peace. Meditation is just one of the components of the HELP approach that will help us break down these walls of isolation as we learn to be more mindful and aware. Meditation can remove isolation by quieting the mind enough to experience an inner sense of peace and well-being that is unifying in nature rather than divisive.

The subtle benefits of meditation may include:

- A feeling of union and integration

- Spiritual attunement

- Inner peace

- Mindfulness of each moment

- Mental balance and equanimity

- Improved concentration

As indicated in previous chapters, the mind is the primary agent in determining our overall well-being. The meditation process is one which allows us to channel the energy of the mind in a positive direction to facilitate the healing process. By disciplining the mind, we can reduce the mental and emotional disturbances and their accompanying physiological responses. This process will allow you to gain that control over the mind through regular practice with a spirit of dedication.

REFLECTING ON THE NATURE OF THE MIND

The mind is often compared to a wild horse or a drunken monkey. It races from one thing to the next, and is very difficult to discipline. Try a simple exercise of just closing your eyes for a few minutes and observing any thoughts or images that pass through the mind. When you have finished, open your eyes and record in your journal what happened.

Now attempt to focus the mind on a single object. Close your eyes and visualize a rose for a few minutes. When finished, open your eyes and answer the following questions in your journal:

- Could you maintain the image of the rose?

- Did other thoughts come into the mind?

- Did other images appear?

- Were you able to go back to the rose?

- Were you aware of external sounds, body sensations, your environment?

- What difference did you notice between focusing on the rose and having no object of concentration?

It only takes a simple exercise such as this to understand the busy nature of the mind. Add to that our daily schedules and the bombardment of sense stimuli during the course of the day, and there is no question that greater control over the mind would not only benefit our physical health but have spillover effects in just about every area of our lives.

Our attention span will be increased and the tendency of the mind to get caught up in the events, words, and emotions that take place around us and leave us feeling unbalanced will be diminished through regular practice of meditation. A sense of greater control, and an ability to be involved in the world and yet have a sense of equanimity in witnessing the events of the mind come and go will allow us to reduce stress and improve the quality of our lives.

How do you feel when you wake up in the morning? The alarm goes off, you get out of bed and go through your morning routine. What thoughts and ideas are going through your mind? Doing the practice of meditation first thing in the morning after fully waking up is an excellent way to start the day with a clear mind, and to develop and deepen the sense of balance. All of us awake and are conditioned by factors in our subconscious and conscious mind, including patterns of behavior that may have been ingrained since our childhood. The meditation process will alert us to this conditioning through enabling us to witness the mental activity, and then to go beyond it.

It is essential to practice meditation regularly in order to gain the physical benefits of a reduction in stress levels and the psychological benefits of greater focus and awareness, with feelings of profound peace and relaxation. All the other components of HELP will benefit from meditation, becoming easier to implement and more effective. Through greater mental concentration and awareness, you will be able to reduce patterns of behavior and reflex actions that may have been detrimental to your overall health, while developing the discipline to substitute the health-promoting techniques of HELP.

Take a moment now to reflect on this basic introduction to meditation and how it can benefit you. Try to understand it fully before proceeding further, and be able to explain why it is important in your overall quality of life. Then think about your current lifestyle and the degree to which the benefits of meditation may enhance your life, whether in your relationships, work, personal health, spiritual development, leisure time, personality issues, conflict resolution, or ability to assist others around you. To what degree could you gain the benefits of the meditation process in any of your other daily activities? Once you have considered this, proceed to the next stage, which will allow you to put this information into action.

PREPARING FOR MEDITATION

Preparing for meditation is extremely important as it will set the tone for all that follows. While we have covered a number of the benefits of meditation, it is best to begin by having no expectations whatsoever, as these will color your mind and will have to be released before any progress can be made. Approach the meditation process in a state of mental neutrality with no fixed agenda of what you desire to happen. By beginning with a commitment to the practice but no anticipated experiences, the mind will be able to proceed through the first two stages—sense withdrawal and concentration—without the obstacles of comparisons and distractions of what is "supposed" to happen.

While you should not become attached to the perfect environment for meditation or any physical objects necessary for you to be able to meditate, if you have a choice, there are ideal surroundings and items which will facilitate the meditation process. For some people these are not possible or even necessary, and you should not let their absence in any way deter you from meditating.

• Try to have a separate area for your meditation which is peaceful.

• Choose a place that is well ventilated with pleasant, low lighting.

• Ensure that you are not likely to be disturbed and the area is as quiet as possible.

- Try to keep the area dust-free, clean, and neat.

- Place visual items in this space that are uplifting to you and positive.

- Have a very quiet clock with a pleasant alarm within arm's reach.

Your choice of location to practice meditation will obviously be dependent on your physical location at any particular time. The more flexible you are in accommodating to what is feasible and practical, the more frequent your practice will become. Physical constraints will always be an easy excuse for not meditating, whether it is because you are traveling, a guest is staying in the house, or whatever the mind chooses to focus on as a deterrent. While you should try to have a regular area for meditation that meets your requirements, remember not to become attached to it, as changes can provide a healthy challenge to your level of commitment. In difficult times many people have had to resort to the toilet or bathroom as the only place they could remain undisturbed for their practice. The regular commitment to meditation is far more important than the insistence on everything being just right. However, if the opportunity to implement these suggestions is there, you will find that a bit of forethought will improve your ability to focus the mind.

Time of Meditation

The best times to meditate are after you wake up in the morning and before you get tired in the evening. The very early morning hours are ideal, and try to do your meditation in the peace and quiet of this part of the day. If you are still sleepy, you may want to splash some cold water on your face, have a shower, or do some stretching and yoga postures to awaken the system. Do not eat before meditation, and in the evening always allow a few hours for your dinner to digest before meditating. It is best to meditate twice a day, and if you start and end your day with meditation, you will establish a very peaceful routine to live by.

Make sure your clothing is clean, loose fitting, and comfortable when you meditate. You may choose to use certain clothes only for meditation which are always available and will cause no discomfort or distraction.

Posture

One of the most important preparations for meditation is your posture. Meditation is available to everyone regardless of their physical flexibility, and can be practiced using any number of different aids to assist you in achieving a position that is both steady and relaxed. You do not have to sit cross-legged on the floor for long periods of time.

The key things to be aware of with your posture are:

• Most importantly, the spine is erect and as straight as possible

• The head, neck, and trunk are in a straight line.

• The chest area is open and well spread out, with shoulders back but not stiff

• The body is steady but not stiff

• The hands and arms are relaxed and resting comfortably

Whether you prefer to sit in a straight-backed chair with your feet on the floor, or cross-legged on the floor, these five guidelines regarding posture apply.

Some people find that it is difficult to keep the spine straight unless sitting in a chair or sitting on the floor with their back up against the wall. Both of these aids are fine. Others prefer to sit on a kneeling stool with their legs tucked underneath the stool, or, if on the floor, to have their buttocks slightly raised by sitting on cushions. Do experiment with a variety of positions at first. Find one that meets the basic requirement of a steady comfortable position which allows you to adhere to the five guidelines. Remember, you want to be able to go beyond your awareness of the physical body, so do not choose a difficult posture that will leave you focusing on tensions in the body during your meditation time. However, we do not recommend lying down on your back, as the tendency in this position is for the mind to begin to wander and lose its focus.

There are several benefits of keeping the spine erect and the head, neck, and trunk in a straight line. It is virtually impossible to succumb to the temptation to fall asleep if this posture is maintained, and the erect spine will help you to remain alert and focus the mental energies on the technique of concentration. As soon as the mind begins to wander or drift off, you may notice that your posture is not as straight as it could be, and that is the time to correct it.

The importance of keeping the chest area open with the shoulders back cannot be stressed enough. The key is to have the chest spread out so that the breath can flow deeply and smoothly in and out of the body. We often hear people say that when we are angry we should take three deep breaths before saying or doing anything, as a way of centering ourselves and calming down. In meditation, the breath is able to become smooth flowing and the rate of respiration is able to decrease as a result of our relaxed state. It is important therefore to allow the chest to expand fully and to avoid the collapsing of the shoulders forward which would restrict the flow of breath.

For many, this posture may seem slightly uncomfortable at first, due to a usual tendency to slouch forward and not have the head, neck, and trunk in a straight line. Do not force too much discomfort onto yourself at once; be gradual, as it is important not to feel stiff in working toward this posture. Eventually the position should be comfortable and allow the body to relax while keeping the mind alert. Work on improving the posture but not in a way that leaves you feeling stiff and distracted. Allow the hands and the arms to relax on the knees or the thighs, wherever is comfortable. Once you have achieved a steady posture, make a firm resolve that you will not move until the end of meditation. If the posture is constantly moving, so is the mind.

The first stages of the meditation process are really techniques of concentrating the mind. Once the mind is concentrated on one point, even the object of concentration will disappear, and the mind will then be in the meditative state. This might take place for just a fraction of a second. However, through regular practice, the meditative state will expand as you gain control of the modifications of the mind.

DEALING WITH MENTAL DISTRACTIONS

There are a variety of options to choose from when selecting a technique of concentration for the mind. They will be considered later. For now, we will look at a key component which is common to all the techniques of concentration: dealing with distractions. First, external distractions (sounds, smells, and so on); and then, internal distractions (thoughts, images, and so on).

Suppose you are waiting in a room by yourself to see someone who is busy at the moment. As you sit in the silence you hear a loud ticking noise from the clock mounted on the waiting-room wall. The ticking of the clock is disconcerting to the point of being annoying. All of a sudden someone you know enters the room and sits down beside you. You begin a conversation. Twenty minutes pass and the person leaves. Sitting alone once again, after reflecting on what was said in the conversation, you become aware of that terrible ticking sound again. It's not that the clock stopped ticking while your friend was present, or your voices drowned it out, because even when your friend left and you were mulling over the conversation you did not hear the clock. What happened was that your concentration was focused elsewhere, and even though your ears were picking up the sound of the clock, your mind was filtering out that input as irrelevant at the time.

We are constantly letting go of sensory inputs to the mind that will distract us from the task at hand and prevent us from concentrating on what we have put our minds to. It is the ability to do this consciously which is the aim of concentration.

When choosing one of the following techniques, remember that the goal is to withdraw your awareness from sensory inputs flowing into the mind, whether they be sounds, smells, or physical sensations. Your mind should ideally become absorbed in your object of concentration to the exclusion of these inputs. Once you have found a technique of concentration that seems to work for you, stick with it. By constantly changing from one technique to another you will not be able to deepen your practice. If you have difficulty leaving the sensory input out of your awareness, begin your practice with a mental inventory of all the senses you are aware of. For example, identify whatever sounds come into your awareness, let them go, and move onto the next. When the mind has settled somewhat, focus your awareness on your technique of concentration.

The next set of obstacles to overcome, after you have moved, to some extent, beyond the senses, is the distracting thoughts, images, and ideas that flow through the mind. These may include memories of the past, concerns about the future, doubts, fears, unfinished business, thoughts of what else you could be doing at that moment, and so on. Do not expect the mind to rest peacefully—it is always a challenge to gain mastery over the mind and make it one-pointed.

There are many ways to deal with distracting thoughts. The first is just to ignore them. Thoughts can be transitory in nature, and as quickly as they come they will also go, if you do not dwell on them. Just return to your object of concentration. If ignoring the thoughts is not successful, there are other ways to handle them.

Acknowledge the distractions and then just let them go. Visualize these distracting thoughts or feelings as leaves falling from a tree and landing in a flowing stream. Always return your awareness to the stream and let the current of the stream carry the leaves away, just let them go. The leaves just flow out of the mind, without getting trapped in it. The stream is always flowing; let it carry any debris of the mind away.

Do not get discouraged by the distractions coming into the mind. When you are focusing your awareness within, it is common for thoughts, images, anxieties, and worries to emerge. Quieting the mind makes you more aware of thoughts that are already there but have gone unnoticed because of your external focus.

Another way to deal with distracting thoughts that still persist is to make a deal with them, as if you were drawing up a contract with the mind—the agreement being that the thoughts leave you alone during the meditation session, and in return you promise to address them as soon as you have finished. Thus you are acknowledging the thoughts and reassuring the mind that you will attend to these things later, but in the meantime you are getting on with your practice.

Some meditators choose to analyze distractions for a few moments as a way of calming the mind. Ask the thoughts why they are coming up now. Let them know that your focus is elsewhere at this time, and ask them why it is so urgent that they be attended to now.

If all else fails in your strategy of dealing with distractions, you may choose to surrender to a particular distraction with awareness. Let that distraction know that it has won, and you will now shift your attention to it. Once you have given in, usually the distraction will disappear and you can return once again to your object of concentration. Remember never to lose your peace over intruding thoughts; that will create two problems out of the one.

In summary, the techniques for dealing with distractions are to:

• Ignore them.

• Acknowledge them and let them go.

• Make a deal to address them when you finish.

• Question them for a few moments as to why they need to be addressed now.

• Surrender to the distractions temporarily giving them a sense of victory.

• Try not to force them out in a way that causes you to lose your peace and become agitated.

Know that your periods of meditation will be challenged but, through your commitment and spirit of adventure, even particularly distracting sessions will pass if you persevere, and this will allow you to experience deep inner peace. If you know other people who meditate, you may find it helpful to meditate in a room with them. This may help you to remain regular in your practice and committed. Group dynamics can be beneficial for all components of HELP, as we all can use a bit of help from our friends.

TECHNIQUES FOR CONCENTRATING THE MIND

There are many techniques to choose from in developing your practice of meditation. Despite what any person or organization may say, there is no technique that is better than any other, although you will probably find one that works best for you. The technique is a tool to help steady and focus the mind. Your full attention upon the object you have chosen is the key, not the object itself. Experiment with the techniques given below, find the one that you feel comfortable with, and remember to stick with the one you have chosen.

There is a variety of techniques to choose from including gentle gazing, breath awareness, and focusing on a sound.

Gentle Gazing

In Integral Yoga, the practice of gentle gazing is also called *tradak,* and involves focusing on any object or symbol that will allow your mind to become focused upon it. Begin by determining where and how you will be sitting. Then place the object or symbol that you will be concentrating on at eye level. This object may be a flower, candle, religious symbol, picture, or anything you choose that will not serve to remind you of your daily activities or concerns. Obviously, if it is an uplifting symbol or object that you hold sacred, all the better. But remember, the object of concentration is a tool to help still and focus the mind, and then to be transcended once the mind is fully concentrated upon it.

E X E R C I S E

Now relax the neck, and move the head slowly from side to side to release any tension. Have the head, neck, and trunk in alignment, with the shoulders back but not tense. Gaze in the general direction of the object you have chosen but do not strain the eyes. Remember not to stare at the object but just gently gaze in its direction. If you find your eyes are becoming tired, close them and visualize the object in your mind as you re-create it. When the image fades, open your eyes once again and resume the gentle gazing. Repeat this process, noticing over time that the fleeting images you see at first when the eyes are closed are replaced by a steady image once the powers of concentration are developed. After a time you will go beyond the image of the object, even if just for a moment, and still have the mind completely absorbed and one-pointed in a meditative state. Do not be in a hurry, and use the techniques listed previously to deal with any distractions that may arise.

When finishing the gentle gazing, close your eyes and use the
following technique to allow them to relax fully. Rub the palms of
your hands together briskly, building up a heat between them. Once
you feel this heat, cup the palms over the eyes, and let the warmth and
darkness soothe and relax the eyes. Once the warmth subsides, stroke
the fingertips across the eyelids a few times, and then relax the hands
and open the eyes when ready.

When practicing gentle gazing, never strain the eyes, and gradually
build up the time you do this practice. Once your powers of
concentration are developed, you will no longer need an object to
gaze at, as it will become part of your powers of visualization.

Breath Awareness

A second approach to concentrating the mind is to focus on breathing.
This practice is strongly recommended, as the breath is always with us,
and it is a very good indicator of our mental state. By focusing on each
breath we can keep our mind in the present moment; as soon as we lose
track of our breathing, we can be sure the mind has become preoccupied
in areas other than the present moment. Take a moment right now to
close your eyes and just follow your breathing for 20 seconds.

The simplicity of this technique is deceiving as it is often just a very
short time before the mind begins to wander away from the breathing.
You may drift off into thoughts of the past or future. You may be
asking yourself why a grown person is sitting with their eyes closed
observing the breath, and thinking about all the other things you could
be doing with this time. You may become aware of a pain or itch in
the body, or any of a thousand other distractions vying for your
awareness. Use the tools listed above to help you let go of these
distractions and return to the breathing.

E X E R C I S E

Close your eyes and become aware of your posture. Begin by
breathing deeply. Slow and deep inhalations and exhalations. The

*mind is following the breath. Forget the outside world and focus
exclusively on the breathing. At this stage do not try to control or
influence the breath; just let it flow naturally and observe as it enters
and leaves the body. You may wish to focus on a particular aspect of
the breathing now. Perhaps the observation of the abdomen rising
and falling as air flows in and out of the body. Repeat to yourself,
"rising," "falling," "rising," "falling" with each full breath. Or you
may choose to bring the awareness to the nose and observe the air as
it enters and leaves the nostrils. Becoming aware of the temperature
of the breath, as it enters the nose in a cool state and leaves in a
warmer state, is yet another tool of breath awareness.*

*If you still find that you are encountering difficulties keeping the
awareness focused on the breathing, you may choose mentally to
count your breaths. By keeping count, we must concentrate on each
breath, which again helps to keep us in the moment. After the first
exhalation count "one." The next time you exhale, count "two," and
continue up to four. After your fourth exhalation, begin again with
one, continuing up to four. When you lose track of the count or
count beyond four, it is a clear sign that the awareness has shifted
away from breathing. Bring the focus back to the breath and start
from "one" again. Over time your power of concentration will
improve, so do not be critical. Just reaffirm your commitment. As
with the mind, so with the body. Make a firm resolution to keep the
body still.*

*A final technique of breath awareness is to tune into the sound of the
breath. Close the eyes, check the posture, and observe the breath,
allowing it to flow naturally. Now begin to listen to the sound of the
breath. If you are careful, you can hear a sound with each
inhalation and exhalation. The inhalation may sound like "so" and
the exhalation may sound like "hum." The sound may be difficult to
hear at first but as your awareness deepens so will your attunement
to it. "So" as the breath flows in, and "hum" as it flows out. Just
stay with each breath and the sound. If the mind drifts away, gently
bring it back to the breath. After practicing this technique for your
allotted time, slowly let the sounds go and become aware of the*

breathing alone, and breathe a little deeper. Then slowly open your eyes when you are ready.

Sound or Mantra Meditation

We are all aware of the power of sound and the qualities that different sounds promote, whether they be a soothing lullaby to help a child relax and drift off to sleep, or the theme song or chant of a sports team to get its supporters revved up. Sound has become a powerful tool in technology (such as sonar or ultrasound) in assisting both navigators and medical personnel. The power of sound can also be harnessed to assist us in the meditation process.

The key is to choose a sound that will help to focus and steady the mind. There is no one sound that is right for everyone, but focus and steadiness are two qualities that whatever sound you choose should promote. It can be a word that has a particularly relaxing effect on you, such as "peace," "calming," "love," or it may be a word or phrase from your religious or philosophical background, such as "amen," "shalom," "Hail Mary," "Om Shanti." The term *mantra* refers to a sound formula often given in yoga teachings as a way of steadying the mind, and it is a common meditation technique in many Eastern traditions.

Choose a word or phrase that works for you and, once you have found one that helps to keep the mind focused and steady, stick with it. The sound that you have chosen will over time become associated in your mind with the qualities of meditation, and will assist you greatly by cueing in the mind to the fact that it is time to calm down and focus the awareness on this sound or phrase.

E X E R C I S E

Now close your eyes, check your posture and take in a few deep breaths. Allow the breath to flow naturally and begin to repeat the word, phrase, or sound. At first you may wish to repeat this sound aloud, and then repeat it silently. If the mind begins to wander once you are repeating it silently, begin to repeat it aloud again. Always train the mind gently to return to the sound or phrase whenever it drifts away. Develop a tempo and tone that promote a feeling of calmness and are comfortable for you. You may wish to coordinate the repetition of the sound with the breathing to maintain a linkage with the breath. When concluding, bring the awareness to the breathing, deepen the breath and when ready slowly open the eyes.

Other Techniques

Feel free to experiment with other techniques of concentration you may read about or be exposed to, but remember that once you find a technique that resonates with you, stick with it, even during difficult times of distraction. Beware of any person or organization who claims that their technique is the "only way" to experience the full benefits of meditation. There are as many different approaches to meditation as there are ways to prepare food. Some people like Italian cooking, others Greek, and so on. Choose the technique that you are attracted to, and generally keep it to yourself as there is no need to advertise it to anyone else. Always remember that the object or technique of concentration will dissolve when you are in deep meditation, so do not get caught up in one technique being better than another, by continually searching for the best or most powerful.

SUGGESTED DAILY PROGRAM

As mentioned earlier, it is suggested that you meditate twice a day, early in the morning and then in the evening. If you tend to have very late dinners, it is perhaps better to meditate before the evening meal, and likewise before breakfast. When choosing the length of time to meditate for, be realistic. Begin by meditating twice a day for 10 minutes at a time. If this seems easy to do, add to your practice in increments of 5 minutes at a time, practicing each increase for at least a week before expanding the time further.

The guiding rule with your daily meditation time is to be realistic. Select a length of time that you are confident you can do daily. It is far better to meditate twice a day for three minutes a session than once a week for a half-hour session. Regular practice on a daily basis is the key to your meditation. You can then slowly expand the duration of your sessions as you become more experienced.

Once you have chosen a period of time for each session and the time of day that works for you, make a commitment to it. Let nothing stand in the way. Excuses for skipping meditation will always be spilling forth from the mind as a way to resist the discipline of the practice. See the games that the mind plays as you develop that internal witness state, and then let them go, remaining faithful to your practice. However, if for some reason it is impossible for you to meditate on a given day, do not give yourself a difficult time for missing your practice. The whole idea of meditation is to assist you to calm and focus the mind, leading eventually to a state of profound peace to heal and repair body, mind, and spirit, which are all intimately connected. If you spend time chastising yourself for not doing your meditation, you will not be promoting this peace. Just make a renewed positive commitment to being regular in your practice. Know that by gaining control over the thought forms of the mind, you are no longer bound by them, and will then experience peace and joy, your true nature.

HELPFUL HINTS FOR PEACE OF MIND

- Establish or join a meditation group.

- Use the HELP meditation audiotape or other meditation tapes.

- Read inspirational books on the benefits of meditation.

- Attend a meditation retreat.

- Record your meditation progress in your journal.

- Take short meditation breaks during the day.

FURTHER READING

Benson, H & Proctor, W. *Beyond the Relaxation Response,* Berkley, New York, 1985.

Gawler, Ian. *You Can Conquer Cancer,* Hill of Content, Melbourne, 1984.

Goldstein, Joseph & Kornfield, Jack. *Seeking the Heart of Wisdom: The Path of Insight Meditation,* Shambhala, Boston, 1987.

Hanh, Thich N. *The Miracle of Mindfulness! A Manual on Meditation,* Beacon Press, Boston, 1976.

Kabat-Zinn, Jon. *Full Catastrophe Living: A Practical Guide to Mindfulness, Meditation, and Healing,* Delacorte Press, New York, 1990.

Meares, Ainsley. *The Wealth Within,* Hill of Content, Melbourne, 1978.

Ornish, Dean. *Dr Dean Ornish's Program for Reversing Heart Disease,* Random House, New York, 1990.

Ram Dass. *Journey of Awakening: A Meditator's Guidebook,* Bantam Books, New York, 1978.

Satchidananda, S. *Beyond Words,* Holt, Rinehart & Winston, New York, 1977.

Suzuki, Shunryu. *Zen Mind Beginner's Mind,* John Weatherhill, New York, 1970.

Creative Expression
AND LEARNING

AREAS OF **HELP** IN THIS CHAPTER

Why be creative?

•

Reflecting on creativity

•

Creativity in action

•

Creativity weekly

H.E.L.P

WHY BE CREATIVE?

Creativity may not be a subject that immediately springs forth in your mind when thinking about ways to enhance your health. Often people associate creativity with the arts, music, and drama, and fail to realize the inherent need everyone has to express creativity irrespective of the form it takes. The denial of this avenue of expression can result in serious impediments to a person's health and well-being through the person's inability to release their unique gifts and, in turn, contribute to the world around them. Instead, a seemingly routine existence becomes a way of life, in which play, excitement, challenge, fun, and risk taking seem to be relics of childhood, inappropriate for responsible adult behavior.

Creative expression and learning are based on a flowing dynamic that utilizes imagination, spontaneity, an element of magic, and self-confidence, without fear of being judged right or wrong in technique. No one taught us as children to incorporate imagination, play, fun, expression, breaking the rules, and learning by doing into our daily behavior. It came naturally to us. Whether in a sandbox or exploring nature, children instinctively create with few inhibitions and then learn about the world through their doing. The HELP program is based on the importance of recapturing these elements within our life. Unfortunately, one of the by-products of growing up is a letting go of many of these elements in life. A notion that they are somehow frivolous, unimportant, and certainly not appropriate behavior unless undertaken in a well-defined area such as sport or drama, is a message that many receive in school and at home.

The HELP program is all about a new message: creative expression and learning by doing are essential components of adult life, even though we may not be aware of their importance. Why be creative? One answer is that it is fun to express ourselves creatively. Another reason is that the universe is in a constant state of change, and this calls for creative responses on our part to situations that may not respond to the same solutions that worked previously. Creativity is a natural phenomenon in a changing world.

Creativity has been applied in the health-care field since human beings first began to take responsibility for developing means by which to heal themselves. From the experimentation with plants and herbs came most of the remedies that are known today. There has been a childlike curiosity as to new and different ways to learn by trial and error without concern of being judged frivolous.

One of the better known recent cases of this creativity in healing was Norman Cousins' foray. A former medical writer, Cousins was diagnosed as having a crippling collagen disease in 1964. Cousins, with the approval of his doctor, decided after an initial stay in hospital that such an institution was no place for a sick man. If he was going to assume the responsibility for battling this disease, he was going to take a creative approach, move into a hotel room, and break the rules. He decided to introduce two therapies for addressing his ailment—large doses of laughter and vitamin C—while at the same time slowly eliminating painkillers and other drugs. Through watching old Marx Brothers' films and classic episodes of "Candid Camera," Cousins observed that 10 minutes of belly laughter produced an anesthetic effect lasting at least two hours, and reduced his sedimentation rate, which indicates the severity of inflammation or infection in the body. Cousins recovered, having reversed what was considered a degenerative and life-threatening disease, through his creative approach.

In his best-selling book *Anatomy of an Illness,* Cousins not only recounts his recovery process but also talks about the importance of creativity. He relates stories of his encounters with Dr Albert Schweitzer and Pablo Casals, and the significance of creative expression in accounting for their health, longevity, and contributions to the world. He concludes, "Long before my own serious illness, I became convinced that creativity, the will to live, hope, faith, and love have biochemical significance and contribute strongly to healing and to well-being."

As time has passed, the creative solution to his disease that Norman Cousins employed has been documented by neuroscientists. Laughter produces increased levels of endorphins and encephalins in the brain:

these peptides act as the body's own painrelievers.

The lesson is not to wait until you are faced with a life-threatening disease to tap into the power of creativity, but to bring it into your life now. While it is not always appropriate to let go of routine behavior, it is clear from the example of Norman Cousins and others that once you are successful in taking a creative approach to life, the very institutions you may be grappling with may find your innovation an effective tool and adopt it. Norman Cousins was later offered a position as lecturer at the University of California Medical School. While it is not possible to prove beyond a doubt that creative expression will increase your lifespan, it most certainly will improve the quality of your life, which will in turn serve to enhance your health.

REFLECTING ON CREATIVITY

As part of the reflection process, take a moment to answer the following questions regarding the role of creative expression and learning in your life, and record the answers in your journal:

- Do you currently have any pursuits that you feel allow you to express your creativity?

- Do you see life as a learning experience in which your sense of play is far more relevant than being right or wrong?

- When asked by a friend who you have not seen for a few weeks what you have been up to, do you respond with any anecdotes that have elements of creativity, or with the same old thing?

- In reviewing your current responsibilities, are you approaching them from the perspective of creative expression and learning with a flowing dynamic, or are you stuck in a set routine and a pattern of problem-solving responses to life?

Your answers will give you a good indication of the role creative expression and learning currently play in your life. If you could lead your life differently, would you choose to inject a degree of creativity, knowing that creative expression and learning are beneficial for all aspects of life? Helping you to answer this question, by putting it into action, is what this component of HELP is all about.

CREATIVITY IN ACTION

If we look beyond the creative arts to aspects of our lives where we would not expect to be engaged in creative expression and learning, the challenge becomes how to be creative in these areas. When examining your work, family, and other daily responsibilities, do you approach them with a sense of creativity, or does routine seem to be the order of the day to help you get everything done? What stops you from approaching these things creatively is the conditioning you have had since school. It is now time to approach life from a slightly different perspective, to allow creativity to flow, to forget about school learning and putting the "right" answer down. It is time to create the reality that you firmly believe in. The following 10 steps may be helpful in stimulating the creative process.

1. Develop a vision of what you want to create.

The first important stage in the process of creative expression and learning is to think about the result you would like to create. For the purpose of this exercise, let's choose to create an enhanced level of health and fitness. You may choose to be more specific than that and focus on a single measure of well-being; the choice is yours as to how specific you want to be with your desired result. Without having a creative vision in sight, it is difficult to focus on creative expression.

2. Examine and evaluate the existing reality.

The next stage is to review the existing situation. Examine the daily steps that you are taking in the area of health from an objective point of view, not getting caught up in what you like to think you are doing but being very clear about what is happening right now. It might be that, with regard to your desired result of improving your health, at the present time you are reading about ways to go about it.

3. See the gap between your vision and reality as the place for the magic of creation.

It is time to take action to bring your desired result into reality. You have a result in mind: health enhancement. You also have a clear view of your current reality: reading about how to bring it about. What you need to do now is to bring the creative process into action and therefore make your desired result a reality. The gap between what you desire to create and what you are presently doing is the playground for the magic of the creative process. Rather than letting it frustrate you, embrace it as the catalyst for your learning.

Creation is all about magic. Having a vision of the desired reality. For a magician this may be sawing an audience volunteer in half without hurting them or breaking free of locks and chains while sinking underwater. Next the magician must deal with the reality of how to create that result, given the fact that saws do cut people and locks are meant to be opened with keys above water. The magic of creation is producing the desired result despite the challenges of the existing reality.

HELP is based on this approach to creativity and learning. There are few people who, when asked in their older years or at a time of physical, mental, or emotional impairment what they would like to create, would say no to health enhancement. Just about everyone would choose to have more energy, have less pain, and feel younger at any time in their life. Once you have made that fundamental choice of what you would like to create, and made a commitment to it, the magic of creativity and learning has begun.

The details of the existing reality may not be clear. People have a way of obscuring reality by seeing what they want to see, or avoiding hard truths in favor of fitting in. The reality in the health area is that first, you as an individual have genetic strengths and weaknesses, and, secondly, given that genetic foundation, HELP offers a range of components that take a creative approach to health enhancement: physical exercise, stress release, food awareness, stretching, quality environment, breathing practices, mind/body connection, service, calming the mind, group support and communication.

The existing reality may be that none of these areas is currently in your life. Perhaps you cannot imagine how you could make your vision of health enhancement a reality given your existing commitments and responsibilities. This is when the magic of creation comes in; when you have a strong belief in the vision irrespective of the existing reality, and a dedicated commitment to bringing that vision into reality no matter what the perceived obstacles. The components that are laid out in HELP are a springboard for this creative expression and learning by doing, not only in terms of health enhancement, but in relation to all aspects of life.

4. Accept trial and error as a given in the process of learning by doing.

This is where the learning process comes in: by experimenting with ways that involve letting go of right and wrong, venturing into new territory, taking a playful approach, releasing the fear of failure, and asking the question "What if I do it this way instead?" Know that all the different paths you take, whether they directly lead to the desired result or not, are part of creative expression through learning by doing.

Creativity is not about achieving the result in the shortest period of time or getting it right all at once; rather, it is about tuning into your intuition. Evaluating and adjusting the process by taking stock of where you have ended up. Then learning from this and carrying on with a spirit of fun, adventure, and challenge, while always keeping in mind your desired result. Perhaps you decide to take up a new sport as part of your goal for healthy exercise, only to find it is not for you. Let it go and venture into new territory.

5. Defy old patterns, logic, rules, the "right way," self-consciousness, and ask "What if?"

When allowing creativity to flow, you begin by disbanding the notion that there is only one "right way" to do something. The duality of right and wrong answers has resulted in blinders being placed on the creative process. When faced with a task, no matter how simple, ask whether there is a way to do it other than how you have dealt with it in the past. When driving the car to a routine destination, is there another "right way" to get there that may present more fun, challenges, or stimulation?

Examine the sacred cows of your right and wrong approaches in life, and experiment by removing these blinders and allowing yourself to learn new ways of doing things, breaking out of old patterns and unleashing a whole new life. It may very well be that the HELP components are not at all mutually exclusive to activities you are already engaged in. That they do not require letting go of other responsibilities and, in fact, may provide you with more energy and time to do more things!

A second limitation on our learning and creative process is our self-consciousness. In addition to there being a "right way" of doing something, there was often a bonus or reward for being right—good grades, praise, monetary compensation, awards—when we were growing up. This not only reinforced the approach but also made the situation of being wrong or different that much more undesirable, with the feared ridicule, failure, rejection, inadequacy, and embarrassment to be avoided at all costs. This self-consciousness has led most of us into patterns of sticking to terrain that is familiar, practical, clear-cut, and follows the rules of the game where the risks are far fewer. It is far less risky to imitate the dietary patterns of those around us than to venture out and create a new way of eating that may expose us to ridicule.

It is important to take a few risks by playing the fool, breaking the rules, veering off into unexplored territory, and not being concerned about how others may view the practicality of these ventures. History is filled with examples of great inventions and contributions that involved people not being afraid to look foolish in their learning-by-doing approach which violated all previous protocols.

Norman Cousins was not the least bit concerned with a possible future as a lecturer at a medical school while lying in bed laughing his way to health with the help of the Marx Brothers. He followed his creative instinct: if negative thoughts and environments contribute to illness, *what if* positive emotions such as joy and laughter were programmed into the healing process? Could they be catalysts for recovery? Norman Cousins took the creative step of asking "What if?" and so began a process of breaking into new territory. Everyone can incorporate the "What if?" strategy into their life, just by asking simple questions that will allow creativity to flow and learning to take place outside of the constraints of being judged crazy.

Neils Bohr, the Nobel Laureate in physics, when responding to a newly proposed scientific theory, was quoted as saying, "We all agree that your theory is crazy, but is it crazy enough?" The Wright Brothers in developing the airplane, Einstein, and many others whose creative genius has changed the world, broke the rules and veered off into new territory with no concern about others perceiving them as foolish. Yet their examples seem to have little effect on most people in breaking away from the crowd, and taking the risk of being judged foolish or frivolous. It is far easier to conform to group and peer pressure than to allow yourself to experience the fun and challenge of creativity and learning by not going along the same old path.

Are current perceived obstacles to health enhancement based around fitting in with the group and being fearful of venturing out to create health in your life?

6. Know you have the power to be creative.

"I am not creative and never have been" is a common response at this stage of the process. Contemplate for a moment the idea that you are creating a reality, which is "I am not creative," and then living it. A self-fulfilling prophecy whereby the denial of your creativity then brings about that reality. Psychologists who have investigated what makes some people creative and others not have found one common denominator: the creative people truly felt they were creative while the others did not. No other factor seemed to distinguish the two groups other than this belief in themselves. It is time to let go of that self-fulfilling prophecy and begin to create. When creating a healthier lifestyle, the key is to know that you can do it.

7. Develop momentum along the way and use it to carry you forward.

There is no better way to help you get over the obstacle of not believing in yourself than to be successful at creating. The key to this is to set small and achievable creative steps on the way to your creative vision. This will allow you to see that you do possess the magic which will carry you forth in reaching your ultimate goal. The importance of building up momentum in the creative process by taking small steps cannot be overstated. When setting goals in your health-enhancement program, remember to make them attainable to allow you to develop this momentum.

8. When stuck, go back to the vision and look at the big picture in relation to the reality.

There will be critical moments along the way when you will require patience, faith, confidence, and a restating of your creative vision to keep your focus. Realizing this before experiencing the feeling of being stuck will allow you to approach that challenging situation with a perspective that will lead to even greater learning. If you focus exclusively on the fact that you are stuck, it is often difficult to find your way out. You could be in the midst of creating a healthier lifestyle and fall ill; remember to keep your vision. Be patient and take a step back. Look at the big picture and you will find the answers to extricating yourself and continuing toward your goal. This is the key to learning by doing when all is not going according to plan.

9. When completed, accept your creation and acknowledge it.

Once you have successfully completed your vision, take time both to accept it and to acknowledge what you have created. In the process of creation the completion of the vision can often be a difficult period. Whatever your creation, take time to acknowledge the fact that you have completed it, and accept all the steps along the way that resulted in it coming to fruition.

10. After acknowledgment, feel the energy being magnified for your next creative vision.

Through this process of completion and acknowledgment, you set the stage for your next creative vision to take place, with the energy reinforced from the creation you have just concluded. By enhancing your own health you may decide to help create opportunities for others to share the benefits of your experience. The creative process will continue as long as you have a vision and a desire to create it.

CREATIVITY WEEKLY

The HELP program is the perfect place to test this approach to creative expression and learning. The vision of enhancing your present health is a goal with which most of you can identify. The creative part is making it happen in your life now. Once you have been successful in this domain, the same creative process is applicable to all other areas of your life. To make it happen now, follow the 10 steps detailed in this chapter:

- Develop a vision of what you want to create.

- Examine and evaluate the existing reality.

- See the gap between your vision and reality as the place for the magic of creation.

- Accept trial and error as a given in the process of learning by doing.

- Defy old patterns, logic, rules, the "right way," self-consciousness, and ask "What if?"

- Know you have the power to be creative.

- Develop momentum along the way and use it to carry you forward.

- When stuck, go back to the vision and look at the big picture in relationship to the reality.

- When completed, accept your creation and acknowledge it.

- Through completion, feel the energy being magnified for your next creative vision.

By allowing creativity to flow into your life you will feel a sense of balance and integration that is beyond description. For those of you who have accepted and acknowledged your creative visions in the past, this experience is a familiar one. For the rest of you, allow HELP to be a catalyst for this experience of creation.

HELPFUL HINTS FOR CREATIVE EXPRESSION

- Use your journal entries as a start for creative writing, drawing, collage.

- Look into local drama, art, music, or other creative-expression classes.

- Look at current relationships, whether at work or home, with family or friends, and let the mind go with creative options.

- Be creative in implementing the HELP components in your life.

- Get together with friends and organize times to entertain yourselves with skits, comedy, and so on.

- When confronted with a problem or feeling stuck, use the 10 creativity guidelines in exploring options.

- Make time to sketch, paint, play with clay, not being concerned about perfection.

FURTHER READING

Cameron, Julia. *The Artist's Way: A Spiritual Path to Higher Creativity,* Tarcher/Perigree, New York, 1992.

Cousins, Norman. *Anatomy of an Illness,* WW Norton, New York, 1979.

Diaz, Adriana. *Freeing the Creative Spirit,* New York, HarperCollins, 1992.

Fritz, Robert. *The Path of Least Resistance,* Fawcett Columbine/Ballantine, New York, 1989.

Kent, Corita & Steward, Jan. *Learning by Heart,* Bantam Books, New York, 1992.

Oech, Roger von. *A Whack on the Side of the Head,* Warner Books, New York, 1983.

Group Support and
COMMUNICATION

AREAS OF HELP IN THIS CHAPTER

Understanding group support

•

Reflecting on sharing and support

•

HELP support groups

•

Establishing a HELP support group

•

Internal communication

•

Communicating with others

•

The art of listening

•

True communication

•

Weekly routine

UNDERSTANDING GROUP SUPPORT

W e are not alone, and we were not meant to feel alone. Despite this, many of us feel a sense of isolation and separation from the world around us at different times of our lives. The causes of these feelings are many: childhood traumas, rejection, failure, ill-health, relationship problems, parental conflict, a spiritual vacuum, confusion, low job satisfaction, lack of self-esteem, unemployment, dormant social skills, retirement, a sense of being unloved, an incapability to share and love, shyness ... and the list goes on. If we take it upon ourselves to undergo an internal search to discover the basis for our isolation, it is possible to estrange ourselves even further from the world around us.

The HELP program is to some extent an individual journey, but this chapter on group support and sharing is perhaps the most important of all. It is essential that this component more than any other be incorporated in your life.

Our lifestyles have undergone significant changes in recent years and, for many of us, feelings of intimacy and interconnection have been a casualty of this process. As the tempo of life quickens, information bombards us, and family and community ties continue to decline, we may find ourselves stranded on an emotional island, with all our thoughts and possessions but no one to share them with. Unfortunately, this is not an exaggeration for many people. Given a continued emphasis on material well-being to the exclusion of spiritual values, an increase in specialization and the use of technology that often leaves us feeling separate, and a decline in viable social, community, and religious structures to take the place of our original village and tribal ancestry, many of us are growing increasingly isolated with each passing day.

If solitude is a conscious choice on your part, as it has been for many great philosophers, poets, and saints, and you feel it is a necessary step to take for your appreciation of the world around you and your role in it, at least you are aware of the consequences of what you have chosen to do, why you are doing it, and you know how to remedy it when the time is right. There is absolutely nothing wrong with periods of solitude; most of our awareness exercises in this program underline the importance of removing yourself from the distractions around you. However, this would be a conscious choice on your part for further development, and this differs greatly from an unconscious drifting away from a sense of connection, leaving feelings of quiet desperation.

Research on the significance and health benefits of sharing and support has been extensive. One well-known study by Dr David Spiegel looked at the effect of group support meetings for women with metastatic breast cancer. Five years later, the women who had met once a week for 90 minutes over the period of one year were found to have twice the survival rate of the control group who had just received the usual medical care. Whether the studies focus on group support meetings, family ties, people involved in community or church activities, relationships and friendships, ethnic and cultural unity, or even pets, the results are impressive. Sharing and support can be one of the best complementary medicines to have at your disposal.

Sharing Our Lives

For most people the thought of sharing their lives revolves around finding a mate with whom they will spend the rest of their lives. In HELP, sharing our lives has a much wider perspective. It involves getting together with people who may be facing a similar challenge to the one we are facing, and sharing our ideas and experiences with them.

The importance of the group dynamic is witnessed time and time again, whether it be with self-help groups that target a specific theme, the team spirit as motivation for sport, or the camaraderie that develops among soldiers during conflict situations to help them through. A shared experience with someone who can relate to what we are currently experiencing seems to resonate deep within our soul, and can begin to break down walls of isolation. Many of us have experienced this nurturing sense of comfort and belonging at some point in our lives, and when we reflect back on that time it can still bring a glow within us. We are social animals, and the key to our physical, mental, and spiritual well-being comes from this feeling of being integrated in body, mind, and spirit with all that is around us.

REFLECTING ON SHARING AND SUPPORT

Take a moment to reflect on the meaning of support and sharing to you. Sit in a comfortable position, close your eyes, and see what words and feelings you associate with sharing and support. Take out your journal now and write down these words and any others that spring forward. Make a full list and, once you have finished, review each word and reflect on whether you are currently experiencing it in your life right now. Perhaps put an asterisk by those that could be enhanced.

When performing this exercise suppose the following words came up:

Intimacy, Openness, Company, Integration, Camaraderie, Larger than Life Itself, Honesty, Compassion, Help, Information Exchange, Community, Love, Balance, Motivation, Perspective

All these things have been shown by research in areas such as psychoneuroimmunology to be very important to our physical and mental health. Most of us would also hold many of these qualities in high regard, yet many of us devote only a limited amount of time to consciously promoting these qualities in our lives. It is as if we assume they will automatically be a part of our lives given our relationships, job, personality, environment, and spiritual pursuits, but this assumption may result in complacency, which will see these things slowly slip away from our lives. We wake up one morning and find ourselves trying to figure out how and why we lost them. We must take time to look at the larger picture, to put things in perspective, and realize that our priorities may not be promoting these qualities.

Go back to your list and reflect on the items you have put an asterisk by. Ask yourself how much time and energy you have put into cultivating these things recently. Record the answers in your journal, and use these reflections as a starting point for your journey of opening up.

HELP SUPPORT GROUPS

Through getting together with others who are participating in HELP, you will receive numerous benefits that will cement elements of the program together. This is one of the reasons that this component of the program is so important. While it may be difficult to organize a HELP support group and to make time in your weekly schedule, know that in the long term the benefits will far outweigh the costs. The benefits to you personally will vary according to what you put into the group and what you are seeking from it; the key ingredients are communication, sharing, honesty, compassion, and forgiveness.

HELP support groups can assist you in implementing the HELP program. The energy that arises from a group of like-minded people can help to foster motivation that you may be lacking on your own in relation to diet, relaxation, exercise, and so forth. You may be able to compare notes with others on, for example, recipe ideas, or how to organize daily life so as to implement the program.

Motivational help and information exchange tend to be the two most frequently thought of reasons for becoming part of a group, yet the benefits can go far beyond these practical matters, to include the establishment of a greater intimacy between yourself and others who may be experiencing similar challenges.

This process of establishing intimacy allows us to realize that we are not alone. That others share similar feelings although the details of their situations may differ greatly. It allows us to gain perspective on our own lives through the shared experience of others. It promotes an openness and honesty among people which friendships and relationships can often mask as we hide behind our images or roles. This sharing can allow a camaraderie to develop among people whose entire link with one another is improving the quality of life, both for themselves and the others in the group. Out of this link can develop a feeling of integration. The individual participants can feel greater through their identity within the group than they perhaps feel individually. They can then use this experience of wholeness to develop their lives so as to take this feeling outside of the group. Most importantly, in this integration process are the two keys of love and fun.

The group may provide an opportunity to develop a sense of humor about your trials and tribulations, and experience the healing power of laughter, joy, jokes, and taking yourself a bit less seriously. Fun is such an important component of life and yet as we grow older it seems to play a smaller and smaller role in our lives. It is as if somehow we are no longer allowed to have fun; it is not appropriate adult behavior. Group support can be an opportunity to usher fun back into your life, through stories, jokes, and looking at the lighter side of even the most unfortunate of situations. The intimacy that group support can create will allow this fun to take place.

The other significant benefit of group support is love: to know that you are worthy of love, and that love can flow through you to others who may benefit from that love. If we could only remember each day to live in a space of unconditional love, most of the other components of this program would take care of themselves. A group can be a place to feel both loving and loved by our fellow human beings, as we go beyond images and roles, and realize that behind them all is a heart just yearning to experience and express love.

ESTABLISHING A HELP SUPPORT GROUP

Following are suggestions that may enhance the quality of support groups. They are by no means rigid and should be seen only as helpful guidelines that you may use at your discretion when becoming involved in, or organizing, a group.

- If possible, secure the services of a facilitator for the group who is experienced and respected by the other members.

- Set up a regular schedule of meeting times and have everyone make a commitment to it.

- Have an agreement of confidentiality. Anything that is said in the room stays in the room.

- Establish common goals and objectives for the group that perhaps are put down on paper and displayed, keeping the focus of the group clear.

- No matter what is said or done in the group, always conclude with a ritual that will allow people to feel a greater sense of unity than when they walked in. A commitment to forgiveness and compassion is helpful when concluding the get-together.

- One of the ground rules must be honesty. The support group is a space where people feel safe to be completely honest and no longer hide behind their roles in society.

When looking at successful sharing in any environment, the key word is communication. Communication skills, both internal as well as sharing with others, are not often given the attention they deserve. To gain the full benefits of group support, consider the following points with regard to your communication skills.

INTERNAL COMMUNICATION

Internal communication is all about knowing ourselves. Before we can communicate effectively with others, we must be clear about our own feelings, and not just what we want to project or think others expect us to be feeling. In order to do this we must take time out for ourselves, and be still. To facilitate the art of internal communication try some of the following techniques:

- Use receptive imagery techniques, meditation, self-inquiry, or just reflection and contemplation. The aim is to be honest with yourself.

- Record feelings in your journal and go over events that you feel are unresolved.

- Become aware of internal conflicts and conflicting priorities that may lie behind your feelings and actions.

- Learn the art of acceptance. By learning to understand and accept yourself the way you are, you begin the process of opening up to growth and development.

- Be honest with yourself about what is happening in your life at this present moment.

We often look outside of ourselves for the reasons we are going through any experience we find ourselves in; we blame external factors, persons, and events when life takes an unexpected turn. It is a similar phenomenon to seeing stress as something outside of ourselves instead of our reaction to change. When we are honest with ourselves, we take responsibility for our feelings. We acknowledge ourselves as the creators of our lives and all the experiences we encounter.

It is also important to remember, when grappling within, to see every challenge in life, no matter how difficult it may be, as a chance for growth and learning. A golden opportunity to take the next step in our understanding and growth. A chance to develop our compassion, love, patience, and equanimity. It is not a matter of blaming ourselves when things go wrong but seeing the opportunity for personal growth in all of life's challenges.

Taking these steps with our internal communication process will then affect our external communication, as we will no longer be looking to blame others, change others, or judge others, but rather just to share our feelings with one another. When you find communication is not happening with others, take a moment to review these points and perhaps you will discover some of the elements for misunderstanding within yourself. It is a shame that our educational system does not train us in the art of communication skills, as they really are the most fundamental skills we can have in learning to live harmoniously on this planet.

COMMUNICATING WITH OTHERS

Realize that everything we say and do each day has implications for whether we will bring a greater degree of intimacy and support into our lives, or isolation and stress. The first thing to remember when communicating with others is the importance of that list you made earlier on sharing and communication. Take an active role in promoting greater sharing with others. By sharing we can open doors that have kept us isolated and have led to misunderstanding. We can assist others who may be experiencing difficulties by simply listening to them. Make a commitment to communication, in terms of both speaking and being an active listener.

THE ART OF LISTENING

The art of listening is a key component of effective communication. How much attention has been given in our education to the skill of being an active listener? Listening is not about second-guessing the other person, and either jumping in with our reactions or mentally switching off, and therefore not really hearing them. Other factors that interfere with active listening include being distracted by thoughts or events around us, a fear of being judged by the other person, being wrapped up in our concerns while another is talking, and not being with that person as they really are in that moment.

To remedy this, try to incorporate the following suggestions when listening:

- Be empathetic. Try to hear the feelings behind what the person is saying. Put yourself in the other's place, and try to feel what the person is feeling.

- Acknowledge what the other person is saying and really hear the person.

- Give yourself the time to listen by being relaxed and open to communication at that time.

- Know that everyone deserves attention and respect, and focus on the positive.

- Be in the moment, right here now. Accept and then let go of fears, expectations, judgments, distractions.

- Establish a sense of equality by sitting without barriers, at the same eye level, with good eye contact.

- Let the person speak without interrupting them with your explanations.

After your next conversation, peruse this list and be aware of whether you need to improve your skills as an active listener. Reflect on the interaction that you had and be honest about whether you exemplified the qualities of patience, being completely with the other person, total receptivity, and a willingness to let them fully express themselves while putting away your own concerns as they spoke.

TRUE COMMUNICATION

When communicating with others, express feelings in preference to thoughts. Feelings allow us to communicate through our heart, and help to bring us closer together. It is important to allow yourself to express what you are feeling. Examine the underlying factors behind your feelings through internal communication, and share them. Our thoughts often reflect judgments or preferences, and may lead us to find solutions in changing the world around us rather than transforming ourselves. Our feelings are real, and honestly express what we are experiencing at this moment.

When a misunderstanding occurs, accept responsibility for your part in it. Be aware that you may have contributed to the misunderstanding through the words you chose, the time you chose to communicate, or a whole range of other factors associated with the conversation. Let go of blame and share responsibility. Remember, the goal is sharing and support leading to greater intimacy. Also be aware of your expectations of the other person. What is it that you want from them as a result of this communication? Put yourself in the other person's shoes so that you are sensitive to their needs.

Let love flow through your communication, both for yourself and those you communicate with. Know that this closeness is really behind your communication and promote it sincerely in your words. When love exists and flows from heart to heart rather than from head to head, true communication takes place.

WEEKLY ROUTINE

While we have focused upon communication, sharing, and group support in general terms in this chapter, it is important to incorporate them actively into our daily lives. Try to make a commitment to the following tasks each week in order to heal the wounds of the past and bring greater intimacy into your life.

• Keep a journal that will promote inner communication using the suggestions of honestly recording your feelings and any unresolved events in your life.

- Try to form a support group, making a commitment to the other members to meet regularly.

- Be aware of your communication patterns for both listening and speaking.

- Regularly go over your list of what sharing and support mean in your life, committing yourself to it.

- Make sure to schedule time in your week for internal communication.

- Remember that the people in your life and you yourself deserve active listening and true communication; so practice the above.

If you forget, embrace unconditional love and have a sense of humor, and all will be well.

HELPFUL HINTS FOR SHARING

- If planning on driving somewhere, always think of someone who might possibly share the journey with you.

- Contact old friends and relatives to rekindle past relationships.

- Exercise with others who you would like to share the activity with.

- Write in your journal and write letters as a way of sharing your thoughts.

- Regularly contact someone who might benefit from having a listening ear.

- Schedule quality time for sharing with a partner or friend in your diary.

- Join or establish a group that reviews books or goes for trips together, or form a group based on your own theme.

- If no one is available, share your feelings with a tree or a flower as a release.

FURTHER READING

Harrison, Dr John. *Love Your Disease*, Angus & Robertson, Sydney, 1992.

Matthews-Simonton, Stephanie, Simonton, Carl & Creighton, James. *Getting Well Again*, Bantam Books, New York, 1978.

Ornish, Dean. *Dr Dean Ornish's Program for Reversing Heart Disease*, Random House, New York, 1990.

Shaffer, Carolyn R & Anundsen, Kristin. *Creating Community Anywhere*, Tarcher/Perigree, New York, 1993.

Spiegel, D, Bloom, JR, Kraemer, HC & Gottheil, E. "Effect of Psychosocial Treatment on Survival of Patients with Metastatic Breast Cancer," *Lancet*, Vol.2: 8668, 1989, 888-890

——"Therapeutic Support Groups," in Moyers, Bill, *Healing and the Mind*, Doubleday, New York, 1993, 157-170

The Art of
SERVING

—

AREAS OF HELP IN THIS CHAPTER

Understanding service

•

Reflecting on service

•

Quality service in action

UNDERSTANDING SERVICE

L ife is all about maintaining balance, and service is a very important aspect of that balance. Of course, we have a variety of needs that we must attend to which often involve taking from the world around us, but in order to balance this taking we must learn how to give something back. True service means that we take time to give our energy to something outside of ourselves with no expectation of reward or payment as our motivation for serving. For some, the art of serving is well ingrained, and this chapter may just be a reminder of things they have learned already but may have lost track of. For others, it will be the first time that they have ever explored the concept of service in their daily activities, outside of the traditional sense of giving someone money to perform a service.

Research conducted on the effect of service on health provides powerful evidence of its benefits, not only for those who are helped, but also for the service providers. One study done by House et al, in Tecumseh, Michigan, focused on 2754 people for up to 12 years. The researchers found that the men who did no volunteer work were two and a half times more likely to die during the study than the men who had volunteered at least once a week. Other research focusing on volunteer work time and again points out the significance of altruism and its positive influence on health (Justice). This is not to say that we serve with the expectation of living longer, but rather that service is an integral part of living. Service reflects a healthy outlook on life, and in itself can help to improve our health further.

REFLECTING ON SERVICE

Begin the reflection by examining your routine, needs, expectations, desires, and disappointments. After thinking about these fully, write down in your journal to what extent these things are based on either serving or being served in one way or another. It is incredible how service comes into just about every aspect of daily lives—in the expectations we have of receiving quality service, as well as in the deep-seated need we have to be able to serve those around us in some form or another. Service is the vehicle for how we express our essence in society. Service allows us to love through giving to others. By serving the world around us, we make tangible the lessons we have learned in life, and contribute to the health and well-being of the planet. We may think that serving others is selfless, but in reality it is perhaps the most selfish thing we do, as it allows us the privilege of giving, to grow, and to feel whole as a result of sharing with others. At the same time, it provides the person receiving the service with both the benefit from the service and the joy of offering someone the opportunity to give of themselves.

We have all experienced periods in our lives when we were searching for the thread of meaning behind it all. Our associations with events outside, people in our lives, emotions within, our state of health: one of these factors took an unexpected turn, and left us feeling in a quandary as to where our life could go from there. Take health as an example; let us reflect on it and see where service comes in.

Perhaps you have just experienced a heart attack, you are in your mid-60s, and you have been advised that you cannot return to your strenuous career without risking further damage and possibly your life. You are sitting in the hospital bed and looking around at all the other patients and the variety of challenges they face. There is a sense of unreality about the whole scene. Yesterday you were active, vibrant, and extremely busy with matters far too important to wait, and with a personal sense of responsibility to coworkers, family, and society. Today you have a sense of despair, as you look around and see so many people clinging onto life, tenaciously battling against the odds. Your ailment, heart disease, is the number one cause of death. More deaths than cancer, AIDS, and all other causes put together! How did this happen to me? What will I do now? Why do I feel so helpless and empty inside?

When you think about forced retirement, there is a void. When you reflect on not being able to run around with the grandchildren without thinking about your heart, there is a feeling of loss. When you think about all the people who have depended on your continued health and well-being, from coworkers to people in society who perhaps did not even know the face behind the service they were receiving, and how this has all changed in an instant, you are lost for words.

Reflect on the roles you cherish in life, that make your life challenging, meaningful, rewarding, and worth tackling. Is there one that does not involve giving or receiving service? Now realize that service provision or acceptance is based on you serving yourself. If you do not look after yourself, all these other areas are in jeopardy.

Service can be divided into four interdependent areas:

• Serving yourself

• Serving other people

• Serving institutions

• Serving the planet

If we neglect quality service in any one of these areas, the whole picture begins to unravel. At times there will be conflict, when serving in one area brings neglect to another—that is where balance and moderation come in—but know that these four areas of service to a great extent will determine just how rewarding your life is. Through quality service life becomes whole, fully integrated, and flowing. What would life be without it?

If you have ever experienced a time when it was not possible to provide any service at all, including the service of receiving (yes, when we receive things from other people we are providing a service, in that we are giving them an opportunity to serve), reflect back on that time. Through this reflection you will be aware of the emptiness it is possible to feel when you are unable to serve in one way or another.

Accumulating money, experiencing life's pleasures, seeking adventure, obtaining power, educating ourselves, having a family, developing a career: these are all masks for the different forms that service takes. Unfortunately, because many of us do not see these things as service, we feel stuck in these roles, until we realize the true art of serving. When we become aware of how important service is to maintaining balance in our lives and allowing us to express ourselves, we can realise the worth of these roles and provide quality service.

Reflect for a moment on what quality service means to you, and write down your thoughts in your journal. Next reflect on this question: how can we serve in a way that will promote peace of mind and ease of body, while being useful to those around us, and experiencing the joy of giving?

We are all familiar with what it feels like to be served, whether in a restaurant or a hospital; we have all been on the receiving end of service. One of the best ways to reflect on the art of serving is to recall a situation in which you were served and your reactions based on that service. The simpler the example, the easier it may be to understand.

Imagine that you go into a restaurant, sit down at a table, and no one comes to give you a menu or take your order. Do you feel a sense of unfairness, neglect, anger, and of course hunger? Of course you do! When you walk into a restaurant, you expect that the people serving will be pleased that you have chosen their establishment, that they will be attentive to your needs, doing their utmost to serve you and make your meal both a delicious and an enjoyable one. In turn, you will respect the restaurant that you are in and its code of conduct. When you are finished, you will pay them fairly for what you have received, and perhaps pass on some feedback, both of which will enable the restaurant to continue to provide quality service in the future. What a beautiful scenario. Then why are you left sitting at this table waiting for a menu and feeling agitated?

A number of circumstances have conspired to teach everyone in the restaurant a range of lessons about service. Five minutes before you walked into the restaurant, the manager received a call from her best friend who had just had a car accident up the road, and desperately needed assistance. The manager gave instructions to the chef to be in charge of all the employees, before rushing out to serve her friend in a time of need. The waiter walked into the kitchen just as the manager was racing out the door. He assumed that the manager was having a break, and that he also deserved a break after a busy afternoon. The chef passed on the manager's instructions to the waiter, but he decided to ignore the instructions and take a needed break. Even though his shift was almost over, it had been so busy in the restaurant in the afternoon that he had not had his full break. The chef likewise decided to take some time off given the manager was not there and he was tired. At that point you walked in and sat down, not knowing any of this.

The chef saw you come in, but it was not his job to give you a menu or take your order; he was there to cook. After a few minutes his conscience got the better of him, and he called out to the waiter in the back that there was someone needing help. The waiter called back that he was on his break to which he was entitled, and that you could leave as far as he was concerned. He had another five minutes, and if the manager could have a break, he certainly deserved one too, as he worked twice as hard on one-third of the pay.

At this point Karl, another waiter, walked into the employees' entrance of the restaurant, 15 minutes early for his shift and looking forward to a quick snack before work as he had not eaten anything all day. He greeted the others and asked where the manager was. Then he noticed you sitting in the restaurant, looking extremely frustrated. He asked the chef whether there had been some type of incident, to which the chef replied it was not his job to know these things.

Karl comes out and approaches you, and asks if he can help. By this time you are ready to explode, and you let him have it with both barrels about how long you have been waiting, and what type of establishment this is. Karl calmly and coolly listens, realizing that he has walked into a dynamic situation that he had no part in creating; in fact, technically he is not even working yet, and besides, he is ravenously hungry. After listening and apologizing profusely, Karl takes your order, offers you a complimentary cold drink, and lets you know that he will do his utmost to ensure that your order is attended to promptly. Karl smiles, and quickly goes back to the kitchen and immediately passes on your order.

The manager, Sue, had walked back into the restaurant just as you launched into your tirade about the poor service, and she heard every word. Sue also comes out to you and apologizes, and decides to share her experience of having to leave urgently to attend a car accident up the road. You had seen the car accident on your way to the restaurant, had thought about stopping to see if anyone needed help, but decided not to because someone else would probably be better at helping. You are glad to hear that everything is okay, and that Sue took the time to do what you had not done. In a way you feel a bit sheepish now about having lost your temper with the waiter. The meal is wonderful, you feel an affinity with the manager and Karl, and promise to recommend the restaurant highly to your friends.

If someone were watching this whole scene from above, a bit like Karl walking into it, they could see the beautiful play of the energy of service being woven into a tapestry. Karl, because of his detachment, was able to handle the challenge, while the other waiter and chef were not. But you and Sue were able to let go of expectations and move on, as both of you were not attached.

QUALITY SERVICE IN ACTION

One of the keys to providing quality service is flexibility, letting go of expectations. This is a form of detachment, not in the sense of not caring, but rather detachment from all the strings we often get caught up in when engaged in providing service. The restaurant story illustrates some of these strings, including:

- Only providing the service that is expected of you when you know more is needed

- Basing your service on what you are getting for it

- Judging others and their service, and then deciding to adjust your service accordingly

- Believing someone else will be better than you at serving, so not providing the service

- Giving quality service only when you feel like you are being supervised

- Ignoring the full implications of not providing quality service in terms of your own needs

If there is one word to describe these strings we get caught up in when providing service it is "expectations." Always be aware of your expectations when providing or receiving service.

- What is expected from you?
- What are you expecting in return?
- What do you expect from others?
- What do you expect of yourself?

If we can let go of our expectations and serve from a place of detachment from expectations, or provide selfless service, we are then providing quality service. How do we let go of these strings and enter into selfless service? Compassion is the answer, not only for serving others but also for serving ourselves. Through compassion we transcend our feelings of isolation and pain, and experience the peace and joy of giving and receiving love with no strings attached.

Following are suggestions to help allow compassion to flow:

- Recognize the needs of those around you by putting yourself in their situation.
- Provide service to those around you without it being contingent on any external reward or acknowledgment.
- Focus at all times on the process of serving rather than any expected result of service.
- Attune to any inner expectations you might still have regarding service and then let them go.
- Try to give more than you receive.

When we serve from a place of compassion, the transformation that takes place on all levels is nothing short of miraculous, because we are no longer caught up in our particular role, but giving from our heart and giving without conditions. An inability to serve or receive service causes us to be isolated and leads to pain and anguish.

How Can I Serve as Part of My Routine?

The beautiful thing about service is that you can do it anytime, anywhere, as long as you are aware of the true nature of quality service.

Some people identify service with charitable or volunteer work. They may dissociate service from the workplace as they are being remunerated for their service. Or they feel that true service takes place beyond the family as there are blood ties and expectations to serve your family. Many people feel they have to go far afield, across the globe, to serve. There is certainly no harm in this, and thank God for those dedicated souls who do it. But let there be no misunderstanding: service is not something that must take place in certain places, between certain times, and under the auspices of specific organizations.

Quality service can be a way of life that you carry with you wherever you go and with whomever you find yourself. It is all about your *motivation* for what you are doing, rather than what others think you may or may not be getting or expecting in return. If you are giving without any expectation of something in return you are providing selfless service.

Whenever possible, using the guidelines noted above, allow quality service to flow into your routine. Let go of expectations and give from your heart in whatever way, shape, or form you are capable of. If you find it difficult at this stage to adopt this attitude in situations where there is too much past history and unresolved emotions, approach community agencies, welfare groups, or people seeking volunteers. Offer some of your time and support in a selfless way. Perhaps if you become aware of serving through these organizations, that same spirit of service will flow into your daily routine wherever you are.

Service is but one component of HELP; it is not to be practiced to the exclusion of other components. It is no good becoming so busy serving others that you do not look after yourself, or you could end up like the man who woke up in the cardiac wing of the hospital unable to deal with his future. Remember to integrate each component into your life; this will then allow you to serve with vitality, humor, and compassion, while remaining healthy and balanced in body, mind, and spirit.

Keep track in your journal of your reflections on the road of serving —the feelings that come up when serving, and the dynamics that take place. Then refer back to the restaurant scene, and the guidelines, to

help to extricate yourself from any strings that may be binding you.
When serving, remember how in your selflessness you are really
being selfish through your knowledge of how quality service breaks
down isolation and pain, and brings intimacy into your life and those
around you. What better way to heal yourself than through serving!

HELPFUL HINTS FOR SERVING

Look in your immediate area for people and organizations to serve. These
may include:

- Family members

- Neighbors

- Coworkers

- Hospice

- Charitable organizations

- Community centers

- The physically challenged

- Religious organizations

- Service clubs

- Prisons

Identify national or international opportunities to serve, including:

- Volunteering abroad

- Environmental campaigns

- Health education and services

- Fundraising for charity

- Hunger and homeless projects

- Peace work

- Human rights

FURTHER READING

Fields, Rick with Taylor, Peggy, Weyler, Rex & Ingrasci, Rick. *Chop Wood, Carry Water: A Guide to Finding Spiritual Fulfillment in Everyday Life*, Jeremy P Tarcher, Los Angeles, 1984.

House, JS, Robbins, C & Metzner, HL. "The Association of Social Relationships and Activities with Mortality: Prospective Evidence from the Tecumseh Community Health Study," *American Journal of Epidemiology*, 116(1),1982, 123-140.

Justice, Blair. *Who Gets Sick: How Beliefs, Moods, and Thoughts Affect Your Health*, Jeremy P Tarcher, Los Angeles, 1987.

Luks, Allan with Payne, Peggy. *The Healing Power of Doing Good*, Fawcett Columbine, New York, 1992.

Ram Dass & Bush, Mirabai. *Compassion in Action: Setting Out on the Path of Service*, Bell Tower, New York, 1992.

Ram Dass & Gorman, Paul. *How Can I Help?: Stories and Reflection on Service*, Alfred Knopf, New York, 1985.

Planning Health ENHANCEMENT

—

UNDERSTANDING PLANNING

HELP is integrative: one or two components on their own will have marginal effect compared with the benefits of combining all components together. The key to the success of this program in your life is to arrange the components into a routine that works for you. This requires a health-management plan that ensures you receive the HELP you need. There are very few people who can alter their behavior and commit themselves to new routines for health enhancement without taking the time to plan how they are going to do it.

Each chapter has included suggestions about how to develop a routine; it is the goal of this final chapter to assist you in interweaving the individual components in a way that is effective, realistic, and enjoyable for you. While it is clear that without health everything else in your life is challenged, it is still important to keep a sense of balance between lifestyle improvements and other daily commitments that you may have. Integration and balance over a long period of time require full commitment and dedication. This approach will be far more effective than a crash course that requires you instantly to abandon habits that are deeply ingrained, and to neglect obligations that you have made and still feel are important. Managing your health requires a plan, which begins with asking yourself why you are embarking on this program.

MOTIVATION

HELP is a comprehensive approach to healthy living which requires you to be clear on why looking after your health is important. Without motivation, all the information and techniques provided will be of little value. Every person may have a different motivation for embarking on HELP. For a great number of people HELP will be a means of dealing with specific health challenges. Their motivation will be to alleviate suffering and regain quality of life. Others will be fortunate enough to use HELP as a preventive tool, allowing them to enjoy life through the maintenance of a healthy body, peaceful mind, and useful life.

Your purpose is your power; define it, develop it, and remind yourself of it daily. Take out your journal and take a moment now to reflect on your underlying motivation for choosing HELP. Ask yourself why you want to help yourself to health. Go beyond the goals you want to achieve and examine the foundation underneath these goals. If one of your goals is to lose weight and you have difficulty addressing the motivation behind it, just ask yourself why. Ultimately, you will find that choosing to lose weight allows you to feel better about yourself, giving you a greater sense of self-esteem. By improving your health, you will feel empowered in many other aspects of your life.

Old habits can be difficult to change. Follow these steps to make your motivational statement meaningful and effective:

- Keep your motivational statement simple.

- Memorize it.

- Write it down in places where you will be reminded of it daily.

- Reflect on how this statement can assist you in other areas of life.

- Develop it and strengthen it by writing these reflections in your journal.

There may still be times when you encounter difficulty in staying motivated despite having followed these steps. To reduce the likelihood of this happening, remember to keep the following points in mind:

- Maintain a realistic approach, avoiding high expectations that are destined to fail

- Whenever possible join in with others to help each of you stay motivated

- Enroll in a class or take on a course of study in a health-related area.

- Refine your motivational statement over time.

PRIORITIES

Begin by revisiting each section of the journal and reflecting on the gap between your existing reality and what you would like to create.

Next, summarize your priorities in the box below, ranking the areas one to 10. There can be more than one component with the same number by it, with one being a very high priority for something currently lacking in your lifestyle, and 10 being for a component that you already have pretty much under control with perhaps some minor adjustments needed.

CHART OF PERSONAL PRIORITIES

Physical exercise

Mind/Body awareness

Food awareness

Meditation

Stress release

Service

Easeful body

Quality environment

Creativity

Breathing techniques

Group support and communication

Planning

SETTING GOALS

Now that you have established your priorities, briefly write down for each heading no more than two sentences specifying a goal for each priority. Remember the SAME rule when writing down the first sentence:

• Specific

• Attainable

- Measurable
- Enjoyable

Making the goal *specific* means that it is clearly understood and therefore easier to make a commitment to. Making your goal *attainable* ensures that you are realistic and not trying to reverse years of neglect overnight. In order to be able to meet your goal successfully, it is helpful to state it in a way that will allow you to *measure* whether you are implementing it. Finally, if you state your goal in a way that is *enjoyable* to you, it will be easier to implement and you will look forward to doing it.

In the second sentence, describe the benefits you will experience in reaching the goal. An example could be:

Physical exercise—*Over the next four weeks, I will develop a daily routine which includes 30 minutes of swimming with Jean and Deborah on Tuesday, Wednesday, and Friday, and walking for 30 minutes with the local group in Eden Park on Monday and Sunday. I will make a commitment to this goal in order to help release stress, improve cardiac fitness, and be healthy enough to enjoy playing with my grandchildren.*

When making your goals attainable, you may wonder if it is possible to fit all 12 components into an already busy lifestyle. As illustrated by the example above, one solution is to combine two or more priorities in the same mission statement—enjoying the quality environment of the park, while sharing and communicating with friends and walking.

It is also important to remember the cost of not looking after your health. Take a moment and reflect on the time that is taken when:

- You are physically sick and out of action from work, from family, from fun.
- You feel tired and cannot finish what you have started due to lack of energy.
- You have an upset stomach and feel distracted by it.

- You are nervous and anxious, and wind up taking twice as long to do a job properly.

- You must visit the dentist, chiropractor, doctor, naturopath, or psychologist, for ailments possibly attributable to an unhealthy lifestyle.

- You daydream and chase after quick-fix schemes that promise immediate transformation.

- You are forced to retire or quit your job due to stress, and use work as the excuse.

- Relationships deteriorate or fail due to lack of awareness, resulting in a long recovery period.

- The body experiences arthritis or pain, and an activity takes twice as long as before.

These are just a few of the many possible consequences of ignoring the HELP components. While there is no guarantee you will not have to see a doctor, or see a relationship fail, HELP is definitely a positive step in all of these areas, and may result in a reduction in time spent dealing with the consequences of neglecting lifestyle factors. The real question is: can you afford to have your schedule overwhelmed by the repercussions of not implementing HELP? The prevention of dis-ease, dis-stress, dis-appointment, and dis-comfort is far less time-consuming than having to live with them, and certainly a lot more enjoyable.

DRAWING UP A SCHEDULE

If you believe that HELP will not only improve the quality of your life but also save you time, then it is important to set up your schedule. You may have already set up this schedule as a result of the routine suggestions at the end of each chapter. If not, now is the time to do so. A well-developed schedule should see you having more time available in your typical day than you had before bringing HELP into your life. The schedule will be a direct translation of your list of priorities and your goals into a timetable format. An example of this could be:

E X E R C I S E

Every day Monday through Sunday

Use the HELP audiotapes, go to a class, or take yourself through a program of one hour every morning, consisting of:

20 minutes stretching and yoga
15 minutes deep relaxation
5 minutes breathing techniques
15 minutes meditation
5 minutes guided imagery.

Balance your meals during the day in accordance with the guidelines you have chosen.

Make sure to take breaks three times during each day for a few minutes at a time to attune within and feel good about yourself, have a laugh, repeat your positive affirmation, be aware of the need for a quality environment, look at a flower, or help someone in need.

Keep your focus by reminding yourself, "In everything I do, I will try to have a sense of humor, a sense of play, take a creative approach, and be positive, loving and forgiving."

Practice 10 minutes of meditation each evening before bed.

Three Days per Week: Saturday, Wednesday, and Sunday

Take one hour of physical exercise—which may be walking, jogging, swimming, cycling, and so on—in nature, incorporating warm-up and cool-down periods.

Thursday Evening

Spend two hours with friends, a support group, sharing and receiving feelings and support.

Saturday

Spend at least two hours in creative pursuits: play, entertainment, sport, drama, music, or any other enjoyable expressive activity.

Sunday Afternoon

Devote one hour to selflessly serving a local community project or perhaps a relative in need.

This timetable covers every component of the program, assuming you are not doing any of them already. Over the course of a week, you have the responsibility of enjoying life and resting for a total of 168 hours. This program, as outlined above, occupies about 18 of them, leaving you 150 hours to do all the other things in life that are important to you. The choice is yours, but just remember that no matter what else you possess, nothing will take the place of an easeful body, a peaceful mind, and a useful life.

ACCEPTANCE, FLEXIBILITY AND INSPIRATION

Let's be honest: this is not the first time we have made a commitment to something that we believed in, and followed all the steps of planning and scheduling, only to find that despite the best intentions the schedule is sitting in a drawer somewhere collecting dust. The key here is to be accepting and flexible.

Sure, you may miss a morning session once in a while due to unforeseen circumstances or the need for extra sleep. Do not despair. *Acceptance* is so important in this program. Help yourself grow through acceptance. Whenever we take on a new venture, we meet with an inner part of us that resists this change. It comes up with excuses as to why change isn't possible and reasons not to change in order to protect its established territory. It looks for contradictions in the underpinnings of the approach to challenge it. It examines the motives of others who may be involved and questions the venture on the basis of these motives. It conspires to upset the routine in any way, shape, or form that is possible, and when all else fails it reminds you of all similar attempts you have made and how you did not see them through. Know that this inner resistance is a part of everyone and accept it, but with the delicacy and agility of a high-wire performer slowly go past it, taking your time and maintaining your balance—realizing that when you fall, the net of acceptance is waiting to embrace you, and that there is really no such thing as failure. As Thomas Edison said, "I have not failed 10,000 times, I have discovered 10,000 ways that will not work."

Also, be *flexible*. Suppose you have been through all the steps of setting priorities, goals, and scheduling, but still find yourself struggling to implement even one of the HELP components. Be flexible in your approach, and realize that at this point in your life perhaps you need to scale down your expectations. Sit down with your schedule and make the changes a little more gradual. When you achieve one, take the time to congratulate yourself, and reward yourself with the praise and appreciation you deserve. Then slowly build up to your previous goals through this flexible approach.

Inspiration is perhaps one of the most important devices to incorporate when attempting to attain any goals. Hearing stories of those who have gone that way before us gives us hope, courage, and determination. Sharing our struggles and commitments with others in support groups inspires us to keep trying. By working together in a group to achieve our goals, we can be inspired by the dynamism of the group energy to go beyond our limited expectations of ourselves.

Do not underestimate the help inspiration can give in accomplishing any of the components of this program. Read books about other people who have overcome incredible odds to achieve major breakthroughs, such as Helen Keller, and let them inspire you in far more modest projects. Let yourself tap into the vitality of the human spirit when challenged, and allow it to carry you to heights that you may never have believed possible. Use pictures, support groups, books, magazines, testimonials, or whatever works for you to inspire action on implementing your schedule. Tell your friends, associates, and family members of your plans and enlist their support if that will help to inspire you. Put notices in prominent places that will remind you of your HELP goals. Use every tool you possibly can to reverse habits that may have been ingrained for many years in order to realize what living is really all about.

THE BIG PICTURE

The beauty of HELP is that when we look after our own health we contribute to the quality of everything around us. We become mindful. We become aware of our actions, and their consequences become more evident, not only in the area of health but in life in general. Our inner attunement is also reflected in our home, workplace, and the environment. We find a beauty and delight in simplicity. Our choices then influence the world around us. A few examples include:

- Breathing practices encourage us to put a high priority on clean, fresh air.

- By choosing fresh healthy foods we encourage those industries to grow.

- Looking after our own health relieves pressure on the health-care system and our families.

- Sharing, supporting, and communicating help to rebuild a sense of community.

- Serving allows everyone to share the gift of life with one another and experience love.

- Choosing a quality environment supports conservation efforts and environmental health.

- Creativity unleashes the imagination and allows it to flow and benefit others.

For each component of HELP there are direct benefits to others and the planet on which we live. By helping ourselves to health, we are really helping one another and the generations to come. May your journey be filled with peace and joy, love and light.

FURTHER READING

Covey, Stephen R. *The Seven Habits of Highly Effective People*, Fireside/Simon & Schuster, New York, 1989.

Frankl, Victor. *Man's Search for Meaning*, Simon & Schuster, New York, 1983.

Gingold, Dr Robert. *Successful Aging*, Oxford University Press, Melbourne, 1992.

McInnes, Lisa, Johnson, Daniel & Marsh, Winston. *How to Motivate, Manage and Market Yourself*, Victoria Cassette Learning Systems, Bulleen, Melbourne, 1989.

Schumacher, EF. *Small Is Beautiful: Economics as if People Mattered*, Harper & Row, New York, 1973.

APPENDIX 1

—

HELPFUL LOW-FAT RECIPES FROM CARLA'S KITCHEN

For quite a few years I was involved in running the Ontos kitchen. I often prepared meals for large groups of people who came to relax and enjoy a new approach to life. The meals at Ontos are all vegetarian, although most of our guests are not vegetarians. Over the years I have had to give a great deal of thought to serving meals that people could recognize and completely enjoy while not feeling threatened by the dietary change. This challenge has brought forth hundreds of recipes and a great deal of information to share with those seeking healthy additions to their diet. The following recipes are just a few of the easy-to-prepare, low-fat dishes that are sumptuous yet simple.

There are a few secret ingredients I would like to mention that make an ordinary meal into a special one. The first of these is to try to develop a peaceful atmosphere when you are in the kitchen. This can be accomplished by playing relaxing music or having uplifting thoughts. Invite family members or good friends to share the experience of meal preparation with you. Secondly, use good-quality organic or biodynamic ingredients whenever possible. Last but not least, use a generous sprinkle of LOVE in everything you make; there is enough love to go around, so use it freely!

TRYING NEW RECIPES

You have decided you would like to incorporate new recipes into your diet. I advise people to start by slowly introducing these recipes. This strategy works well for those who would like to share these meals with family members who may be reluctant to change. You could begin by preparing one or two new recipes a week; do this for a few weeks, then make three or four a week until you are satisfied with the change. If you are following a low-fat diet or would like to reduce your fat intake, you can use this same method to cut down gradually on dairy products and oils. Do not be discouraged if the new dishes you try do not turn out the first time—practice makes perfect. I would also like to encourage you to use your initiative and imagination and experiment with your own ideas.

ADAPTING RECIPES

I love cookbooks and if you are anything like me you probably have a shelf full. Cookbooks are easy, light, good-fun reading and can be a source of inspiration on those days when you just cannot think of what to make. Any cookbook is still of good use even if you have chosen to follow a low-fat or vegetarian diet. Recipes can be adapted simply by removing the meat and replacing it with one or a combination of the following:

For casseroles and stews:

• Grains (cooked millet, rice, burghul, and quinoa)

• Beans (cooked red kidney beans, soya, haricot, black eye, and borlotti—cranberry beans)

• Legumes (lentils—red and green or brown, cooked garbanzo, or chickpeas)

• Beancurd (tofu)—fresh crumbled, or frozen then defrosted

In sauces and stews:

• Beancurd (tofu)—fresh crumbled, or frozen then defrosted

• Vegetables, finely diced (carrots, squash, onions, mushrooms, and celery)

Dressings instead of oil:

• Non-fat yogurt

• Beancurd (tofu)

- Tomato juice

- A little mustard for extra flavor

Many recipes ask for sautéing with oil or butter, simply cook in about half a cup of water or vegetable broth instead. This does not compromise flavor, although foods are not as rich. Try experimenting with herbs and spices. Your only restriction is your imagination and that is unlimited. Be adventurous and enjoy your new journey to health.

SOUPS

Pumpkin Soup

1 medium-size butternut pumpkin, peeled and chopped into small pieces

1 medium onion, finely chopped

2 cloves garlic, finely chopped

$\frac{1}{4}$ teaspoon nutmeg

1 vegetable stock cube

parsley to taste, chopped

chives to taste, chopped

1. Place all the ingredients in a large saucepan and cover with water. Bring to the boil and simmer until cooked (about 30 minutes).

2. Place the soup in a food processor and blend to a smooth consistency.

3. Return to the saucepan and reheat.

4. Serve garnished with the parsley and chives.

Variations: Substitute potato for half of the pumpkin.
   Use leek instead of onion.

Red Lentil Soup

2 cups red lentils, washed

1½ cups carrot, grated

1 stick celery, finely sliced

1 medium onion, finely diced

1 vegetable stock cube

2 large bay leaves

½ cup parsley, chopped

1. Place all the ingredients except the parsley in a large saucepan, and bring to the boil. Allow to simmer until cooked (about 30 minutes).

2. Remove the bay leaves, then place the soup in a food processor and blend until smooth.

3. Reserve some of the parsley for garnish, and add the remaining parsley to the soup.

4. Return to the saucepan and cook for another 10 minutes.

5. Serve garnished with the reserved parsley.

Vegetable Soup

1 medium onion, finely diced

1 medium carrot, finely diced

2 stalks celery, finely sliced

1 medium potato, finely diced

1 medium tomato, roughly chopped (optional)

1 small swiss chard (silver beet) leaf, finely shredded

1 cup of asparagus, $1/2$ cup broccoli, and $1/2$ cup cauliflower, or any other combination of vegetables you may enjoy

1 vegetable stock cube

$1/2$ cup parsley, finely chopped

1. Reserving some of the parsley for garnish, place all the ingredients in a large saucepan and cover with water (the water should cover the vegetables by about $1^1/_4$ in, or 4 cm). Bring to the boil and allow to simmer for 20–30 minutes.

2. Serve garnished with the reserved parsley.

MAIN MEALS

Beancurd (Tofu) and Zucchini Quiche

1 large onion, finely diced

2 cups zucchini, grated and squeezed

2 cloves garlic, finely chopped or grated

$\frac{1}{2}$ cup parsley, finely chopped

1 tbsp fresh basil, finely chopped, or 1 tsp dry

1 block beancurd (tofu), blended until fairly smooth

$1\frac{1}{2}$ tbsps tamari to taste

1. In a large frying pan, cook the onion in about $\frac{1}{2}$ cup of water until transparent.

2. Add the zucchini, garlic, parsley, and basil, and cook a little longer.

3. Tip this mixture into a large mixing bowl and combine with the beancurd and tamari.

4. Pour the beancurd mixture into a baking dish oiled or unoiled and bake in a 180°C (355°F) oven for 1 hour or until it sets.

5. Serve.

Beancurd (Tofu) Burgers

1 block beancurd (tofu), mashed

2 cloves garlic, finely chopped or grated

$\frac{1}{2}$ cup parsley

$\frac{1}{2}$ cup celery plus leaves, finely chopped

$1\frac{1}{2}$ tsps curry powder of your choice

$\frac{1}{2}$ cup tamari

2 cups cooked millet, or rolled oats on the dry side, or rice, or bread crumbs, or matza meal

1 cup plain flour, or flour and cornmeal (polenta)

1. Combine all the ingredients together in a large mixing bowl. Believe it or not, your hands are the best utensils for this step. You need to squash and knead the mixture so that it binds together well. It should look like a wet but firm dough.

2. Place the flour, or flour and cornmeal mixture, in another mixing bowl. Shape the mixture into burgers the size of golf balls, roll the burgers in the flour or flour mix, then flatten to $\frac{3}{8}$ in (1 cm) rounds. (To stop the mixture from sticking to your hands, have a bowl of water by you so that you can dip your hands in between rolling each burger.)

3. Place the burgers on an oiled baking tray and bake at 180°C (355°F) for 15–20 minutes.

4. Serve with hot tomato sauce, mustard or chutney in a healthy bread roll with lettuce, tomato or beets.

Mexican Beans

1 cup onion, finely diced

2 cloves garlic, finely chopped or grated

1 tbsp cumin

3 cups cooked pinto beans, red kidney beans or borlotti beans

1 cup cooking water from the beans

1 cup potato, mashed

$\frac{1}{2}$ vegetable stock cube

12 taco shells

Salad vegetables: lettuce, tomato, cucumber, bell pepper (capsicum), onion

1. In a medium frying pan, cook the onion in about $\frac{1}{2}$ cup of water until transparent. Add the garlic and cumin, and cook for about 1 minute longer.

2. Transfer to a large saucepan and add the beans, potato, and stock cube. Cover with the cooking water and simmer for 15 minutes, or until the beans are mushy. The mixture should resemble a thick paste.

3. While the mixture is cooking, place the taco shells in a low oven to warm. Shred the lettuce, slice the tomato and cucumber, and dice the bell pepper and onion.

4. To serve, place the cooked bean mixture along with the salad vegetables in the warmed taco shells. Have some Hot Tomato Sauce on hand (see page 185).

Lima Bean Casserole

1 large onion, diced

$\frac{1}{2}$ cup celery, sliced

1 cup carrot, diced

$\frac{1}{2}$ cup sweet potato, diced

2 cloves garlic

$\frac{1}{2}$ cup parsley, chopped

2 bay leaves

1 tsp dried oregano, or 1 tbsn fresh, chopped

1 vegetable stock cube

2 cups water

2 cups cooked lima beans (approximately 1 cup raw cooks up to this amount)

1 tbsp cornstarch (cornflour)

1. In a large frying pan, cook the onion in about $\frac{1}{2}$ cup of water until transparent. Add the celery, carrot, sweet potato, garlic, and herbs, and cook a little longer.

2. Transfer to a large lidded saucepan, add 1 cup of water, the stock cube, and the beans, and allow to simmer with the lid on for a few minutes.

3. Mix the cornstarch with remaining cold water and add to the vegetables as you stir.

4. Remove from the heat and pour into a casserole dish. Bake for 30 minutes at 180°C (355°F).

Variation: Use mashed potato on top.

SIDE DISHES

Herb Baked Potatoes

6 medium red or white potatoes

2 tbsps fresh rosemary leaves, roughly cut

2 tbsps fresh sage leaves, roughly cut

1. Cut the potatoes into small pieces, place into a baking dish with $\frac{1}{2}$ cup of water, and sprinkle with the herbs.

2. Bake at 200°C (400°F) until cooked. (The time depends on the size of the potatoes.) You may need to add more water at intervals so that the potatoes don't stick to the bottom of the baking dish.

3. Serve hot.

Mushroom Rice

1 onion, thinly sliced

3 cups mushrooms, thinly sliced

3 cloves garlic, finely chopped or grated

$1\frac{1}{2}$ cups whole brown rice

1 vegetable stock cube

1 cup parsley

1. In a large lidded frying pan, cook the onion in about $\frac{1}{2}$ cup of water until transparent. Add the mushrooms and garlic, cover and continue to cook until all the water is absorbed. Stir occasionally.

2. Transfer to a large lidded saucepan, add the rice, stock cube and 3 cups of water. Cover and simmer until the rice is cooked.

3. Serve garnished with the parsley.

Hot Tomato Sauce

1 medium onion, finely diced

2 cloves garlic, finely chopped or grated

1 medium bell pepper (capsicum), finely diced (optional)

1 large tomato, chopped

1 can of tomato puree

$^1/_2$ tsp cayenne pepper, or to taste

$^1/_2$ vegetable stock cube, or salt and pepper to taste

1. In a large saucepan, cook the onion in about $^1/_2$ cup of water until transparent.

2. Add the rest of the ingredients, cover and allow to simmer for about 20 minutes.

3. Serve as an accompaniment to Mexican Beans, pasta dishes, baked potatoes or anything you enjoy with tomato sauce.

DESSERTS

Healthy Ice cream

Freeze your favorite fruit in small pieces, and when it is frozen blend it in a food processor or blender. Suitable fruits that I have tried are bananas, strawberries, apricots, peaches, raspberries, papaya (papaw), kiwis (Kiwi fruit), or a combination of these.

Variation: Use 1 part fruit and 1 part frozen soya milk.

Soya Milk Rice Custard

2 cups cooked rice

½ cup sultanas, soaked for 1 hour or longer

2 cups soya milk

½ cup dates, soaked overnight and blended

¼ cup honey

1. Place the rice in a baking dish.
2. In a food processor, blend the sultanas with half the milk. Add the dates, the rest of the milk and the honey, and stir the mixture through the rice.
3. Bake at 180°C (355°F) until firm (about 40 minutes).
4. Serve hot or cold

Ricotta and Fruit Pudding

$^1/_2$ cup dried pitted prunes

$^1/_2$ cup dried apricots (optional)

water or your favorite fruit juice

1 lb (500 g) ricotta cheese

$^1/_4$ cup blackberry, or your favorite, jam

$^1/_2$ tsp vanilla extract

1. Soak the dried fruit overnight in enough water or fruit juice to
   cover. Drain, then cut into pieces and set aside.
2. Place the ricotta in a food processor and blend until quite light and
   creamy. Add the jam and vanilla extract and blend a little longer.
3. Transfer to a mixing bowl and fold in the fruit.
4. Serve the pudding by itself, with fruit salad, or as filling for an
   uncooked cheesecake.

BREAKFAST

Baked Millet

1 cup ground millet

Note: Millet goes rancid easily when ground and exposed to light, so it's best to buy whole hulled millet and grind it as you need it, in a seed grinder. It will taste very bitter if it is rancid.

1. In a large saucepan, bring 3 cups of water to the boil, and whisk in the millet. Cover and bring to the boil again.

2. Remove from the heat and pour into a baking dish. Cover and bake for 20 minutes at 180°C (355°F).

3. Serve hot.

Variations: Add ½ cup of ripe banana and ½ cup of dates, or ½ cup of prunes before baking.

Quick Rolled Oats

2 cups biodynamic rolled oats

½ cup dried fruit (optional)

1. Soak the rolled oats in 2 cups of water overnight. If you would like to use dried fruit in this recipe, soak them with the rolled oats.

2. In the morning bring the porridge to the boil, then simmer for 5 minutes, stirring constantly.

Neal's Fruit Salad

3 cups apple juice or orange juice

1 apple, cored and diced

2 ripe bananas, sliced

$1/4$ ripe pineapple, cored and cut into chunks

4 kiwis (Kiwi fruit), peeled and sliced

1 orange, peeled, cut in half lengthwise and sliced

1 mandarin, peeled and sectioned

1 pear, cored and cut into pieces

$1/4$ cup sultanas

$1/4$ cup currants

A few sprigs of mint

Combine all the ingredients together and garnish with the mint.

APPENDIX 2

—

A JOURNAL TO HELP YOURSELF TO HEALTH

If you have built castles in the air, your work need not be lost; that is where they should be. Now put the foundations under them.

– HENRY DAVID THOREAU

The pages that follow are designed to get you started with your journal. To begin, photocopy the pages and use them to start each of the 12 sections of your HELP journal. Answer the questions in the reflection section of each chapter on these pages, as well as your responses from Chapter 12 on motivation, priorities and goals. Place plenty of blank pages in each section in order to expand, update, and revise your goals, reflections, and schedules as the HELP journey proceeds.

Remember to allow your journal to be a creative exercise and feel free to include drawings, photos, objects from nature, cartoons, or anything else that comes to mind. Do not let your writing style or lack of practice inhibit you; just pick up a pen and let whatever you are feeling or thinking flow onto the page. Take a moment to read the quotes at the start of each section for reminders and inspiration.

Enjoy your journal and treat it as a friend with whom you can share your feelings and grow. Take time to read your journal to remind yourself of the progress you have made. You will find this particularly useful when encountering difficulties and feeling a little low on motivation.

HELPFUL REFLECTIONS ON

Chapter 1

RELEASING STRESS

—

*First keep the peace within yourself, then you can also
bring peace to others.*

—THOMAS À KEMPIS

Today's Date: **Time:**   **Location:**

Write a few words describing how you feel right now:

_____

_____

_____

_____

_____

Your answers to questions from the reflection section of Chapter 1:

_____

_____

_____

_____

_____

Your motivation statement from Chapter 12:

_____

_____

_____

_____

_____

How high a priority is stress release on your chart of personal
priorities from Chapter 12?

_____

Write two sentences that clearly state your goal for stress release,
which is _specific, attainable, measurable,_ and _enjoyable:_

_____

_____

_____

_____

_____

_____

_____

From this page forward, regularly enter updates on releasing stress by
adding your own pages. Keep track of your reflections, progress,
goals, and daily schedule, using a similar layout as displayed at the
top of the opposite page. Be accepting of challenges and disruptions.
Be flexible in your implementation schedule. Maintain your
inspiration by working with others, reading, reflecting, and reminding
yourself of your motivation statement.

HELPFUL REFLECTIONS ON

Chapter 2

PHYSICAL EXERCISE

___

Those who think they have not time for bodily exercise will sooner or later have to find time for illness.

—EDWARD STANLEY, 15TH EARL OF DERBY

Today's Date: **Time:**   **Location:**

Write a few words describing how you feel right now:

_____

_____

_____

_____

_____

Your answers to questions from the reflection section of Chapter 2:

_____

_____

_____

_____

_____

Your motivation statement from Chapter 12:

_____

_____

_____

_____

_____

How high a priority is physical exercise on your chart of personal
priorities from Chapter 12?

_____

Write two sentences that clearly state your goal for physical exercise,
which is *specific, attainable, measurable,* and *enjoyable:*

_____

_____

_____

_____

_____

_____

_____

_____

From this page forward, regularly enter updates on physical exercise
by adding your own pages. Keep track of your reflections, progress,
goals, and daily schedule, using a similar layout as displayed at the
top of the opposite page. Be accepting of challenges and disruptions.
Be flexible in your implementation schedule. Maintain your
inspiration by working with others, reading, reflecting, and reminding
yourself of your motivation statement.

HELPFUL REFLECTIONS ON

Chapter 3

AN EASEFUL BODY

—

Our bodies are our gardens, to which our wills are gardeners.

—WILLIAM SHAKESPEARE

Today's Date: **Time:**   **Location:**

Write a few words describing how you feel right now:

_____

_____

_____

_____

_____

Your answers to questions from the reflection section of Chapter 3:

_____

_____

_____

_____

_____

Your motivation statement from Chapter 12:

_____

_____

_____

_____

_____

How high a priority is an easeful body on your chart of personal
priorities from Chapter 12?

_____

Write two sentences that clearly state your goal for an easeful body,
which is *specific, attainable, measurable,* and *enjoyable:*

_____

_____

_____

_____

_____

_____

_____

_____

From this page forward, regularly enter updates on an easeful body by
adding your own pages. Keep track of your reflections, progress,
goals, and daily schedule, using a similar layout as displayed at the
top of the opposite page. Be accepting of challenges and disruptions.
Be flexible in your implementation schedule. Maintain your
inspiration by working with others, reading, reflecting, and reminding
yourself of your motivation statement.

HELPFUL REFLECTIONS ON

Chapter 4

A QUALITY ENVIRONMENT

The frog does not drink up the pond in which he lives.

—BUDDHIST PROVERB

Today's Date: **Time:**   **Location:**

Write a few words describing how you feel right now:

_____

_____

_____

_____

Your answers to questions from the reflection section of Chapter 4:

_____

_____

_____

_____

Your motivation statement from Chapter 12:

_____

_____

_____

_____

How high a priority is a quality environment on your chart of personal priorities from Chapter 12?

_____

Write two sentences that clearly state your goal for a quality environment, which is *specific, attainable, measurable,* and *enjoyable:*

_____

_____

_____

_____

_____

_____

_____

From this page forward, regularly enter updates on a quality environment by adding your own pages. Keep track of your reflections, progress, goals, and daily schedule, using a similar layout as displayed at the top of the opposite page. Be accepting of challenges and disruptions. Be flexible in your implementation schedule. Maintain your inspiration by working with others, reading, reflecting, and reminding yourself of your motivation statement.

HELPFUL REFLECTIONS ON

Chapter 5

FOOD AWARENESS

■

You put a baby in a crib with an apple and a rabbit. If it eats the rabbit and plays with the apple, I'll buy you a new car.

–HARVEY DIAMOND

Today's Date: **Time:**   **Location:**

Write a few words describing how you feel right now:

_____

_____

_____

_____

_____

Your answers to questions from the reflection section of Chapter 5:

_____

_____

_____

_____

_____

Your motivation statement from Chapter 12:

_____

_____

_____

_____

_____

How high a priority is food awareness on your chart of personal
priorities from Chapter 12?

_____

Write two sentences that clearly state your goal for food awareness,
which is *specific, attainable, measurable,* and *enjoyable:*

_____

_____

_____

_____

_____

_____

_____

_____

From this page forward, regularly enter updates on food awareness by
adding your own pages. Keep track of your reflections, progress,
goals, and daily schedule, using a similar layout as displayed at the
top of the opposite page. Be accepting of challenges and disruptions.
Be flexible in your implementation schedule. Maintain your
inspiration by working with others, reading, reflecting, and reminding
yourself of your motivation statement.

HELPFUL REFLECTIONS ON

Chapter 6

THE MIND/BODY CONNECTION

—

Laughter is inner jogging.

—NORMAN COUSINS

Today's Date: **Time:**   **Location:**

Write a few words describing how you feel right now:

_____

_____

_____

_____

Your answers to questions from the reflection section of Chapter 6:

_____

_____

_____

_____

Your motivation statement from Chapter 12:

_____

_____

_____

_____

_____

How high a priority is mind/body awareness on your chart of personal
priorities from Chapter 12?

_____

Write two sentences that clearly state your goal for mind/body
awareness, which is *specific, attainable, measurable,* and *enjoyable:*

_____

_____

_____

_____

_____

_____

_____

From this page forward, regularly enter updates on mind/body
awareness by adding your own pages. Keep track of your reflections,
progress, goals, and daily schedule, using a similar layout as
displayed at the top of the opposite page. Be accepting of challenges
and disruptions. Be flexible in your implementation schedule.
Maintain your inspiration by working with others, reading, reflecting,
and reminding yourself of your motivation statement.

HELPFUL REFLECTIONS ON

Chapter 7

BREATH OF LIFE

———

There's only one corner of the universe you can be
certain of improving and that's your own self.

—ALDOUS HUXLEY

Today's Date: **Time:**   **Location:**

Write a few words describing how you feel right now:

_____

_____

_____

_____

_____

Your answers to questions from the reflection section of Chapter 7:

_____

_____

_____

_____

_____

Your motivation statement from Chapter 12:

_____

_____

_____

_____

How high a priority is using breathing techniques on your chart of
personal priorities from Chapter 12?

_____

Write two sentences that clearly state your goal for using breathing
techniques, which is _specific, attainable, measurable,_ and _enjoyable:_

_____

_____

_____

_____

_____

_____

_____

From this page forward, regularly enter updates on using breathing
techniques by adding your own pages. Keep track of your reflections,
progress, goals and daily schedule, using a similar layout as displayed
at the top of the opposite page. Be accepting of challenges and
disruptions. Be flexible in your implementation schedule. Maintain
your inspiration by working with others, reading, reflecting, and
reminding yourself of your motivation statement.

HELPFUL REFLECTIONS ON

Chapter 8

A PEACEFUL MIND

———

Flow with whatever may happen and let your mind be free. Stay centered by accepting whatever you are doing. This is the ultimate.

—CHUANG TSU

Today's Date: **Time:**   **Location:**

Write a few words describing how you feel right now:

_____

_____

_____

_____

_____

Your answers to questions from the reflection section of Chapter 8:

_____

_____

_____

_____

_____

Your motivation statement from Chapter 12:

_____

_____

_____

_____

How high a priority is meditation on your chart of personal priorities from Chapter 12?

_____

Write two sentences that clearly state your goal for meditating, which is *specific, attainable, measurable,* and *enjoyable:*

_____

_____

_____

_____

_____

_____

_____

From this page forward, regularly enter updates on meditation by adding your own pages. Keep track of your reflections, progress, goals, and daily schedule, using a similar layout as displayed at the top of the opposite page. Be accepting of challenges and disruptions. Be flexible in your implementation schedule. Maintain your inspiration by working with others, reading, reflecting, and reminding yourself of your motivation statement.

HELPFUL REFLECTIONS ON

Chapter 9

CREATIVE EXPRESSION AND LEARNING

—

Imagination is more important than knowledge.

—ALBERT EINSTEIN

Today's Date: **Time:**   **Location:**

Write a few words describing how you feel right now:

_____

_____

_____

_____

_____

Your answers to questions from the reflection section of Chapter 9:

_____

_____

_____

_____

_____

Your motivation statement from Chapter 12:

_____

_____

_____

_____

_____

How high a priority is creativity on your chart of personal priorities
from Chapter 12?

_____

Write two sentences that clearly state your goal for creativity, which is
specific, attainable, measurable, and *enjoyable:*

_____

_____

_____

_____

_____

_____

_____

_____

From this page forward, regularly enter updates on creativity by
adding your own pages. Keep track of your reflections, progress,
goals, and daily schedule, using a similar layout as displayed at the
top of the opposite page. Be accepting of challenges and disruptions.
Be flexible in your implementation schedule. Maintain your
inspiration by working with others, reading, reflecting, and reminding
yourself of your motivation statement.

HELPFUL REFLECTIONS ON

Chapter 10

GROUP SUPPORT AND COMMUNICATION

——

It is one of the most beautiful compensations of this life that no man can sincerely try to help another without helping himself...

–RALPH WALDO EMERSON

Today's Date: **Time:**   **Location:**

Write a few words describing how you feel right now:

_____

_____

_____

_____

_____

Your answers to questions from the reflection section of Chapter 10:

_____

_____

_____

_____

_____

Your motivation statement from Chapter 12:

_____

_____

_____

_____

_____

How high a priority is group support and communication on your
chart of personal priorities from Chapter 12?

_____

Write two sentences that clearly state your goal for group support and
communication, which is *specific, attainable, measurable,* and
enjoyable:

_____

_____

_____

_____

_____

_____

_____

_____

From this page forward, regularly enter updates on group support and
communication by adding your own pages. Keep track of your
reflections, progress, goals, and daily schedule, using a similar layout
as displayed at the top of the opposite page. Be accepting of
challenges and disruptions. Be flexible in your implementation
schedule. Maintain your inspiration by working with others, reading,
reflecting, and reminding yourself of your motivation statement.

HELPFUL REFLECTIONS ON

Chapter 11

THE ART OF SERVING

*Small service is true service. The daisy, by the shadow
that it casts, protects the lingering dewdrop from the sun.*

—WILLIAM WORDSWORTH

Today's Date: **Time:**   **Location:**

Write a few words describing how you feel right now:

_____

_____

_____

_____

_____

Your answers to questions from the reflection section of Chapter 11:

_____

_____

_____

_____

_____

Your motivation statement from Chapter 12:

_____

_____

_____

_____

_____

How high a priority is service on your chart of personal priorities
from Chapter 12?

_____

Write two sentences that clearly state your goal for service, which is
specific, attainable, measurable, and *enjoyable:*

_____

_____

_____

_____

_____

_____

_____

_____

From this page forward, regularly enter updates on service by adding
your own pages. Keep track of your reflections, progress, goals, and
daily schedule, using a similar layout as displayed at the top of the
opposite page. Be accepting of challenges and disruptions. Be flexible
in your implementation schedule. Maintain your inspiration by
working with others, reading, reflecting, and reminding yourself of
your motivation statement.

HELPFUL REFLECTIONS ON

Chapter 12

PLANNING HEALTH ENHANCEMENT

——

Whatever you can do or dream you can do, begin it.
Boldness has genius, power and magic to it.

–JOHANN WOLFGANG VON GOETHE

Today's Date: **Time:**   **Location:**

Write a few words describing how you feel right now:

_____

_____

_____

_____

_____

Your answers to questions from the reflection section of Chapter 12:

_____

_____

_____

_____

Your motivation statement from Chapter 12:

_____

_____

_____

How high a priority is planning on your chart of personal priorities from Chapter 12?

_____

Write two sentences that clearly state your goal for planning, which is _specific, attainable, measurable,_ and _enjoyable:_

_____

_____

_____

_____

_____

Write down your weekly schedule that you have planned for all your HELP priorities:

_____

_____

_____

_____

_____

From this page forward, regularly enter updates on planning by adding your own pages. Keep track of your reflections, progress, goals, and daily schedule, using a similar layout as displayed at the top of the opposite page. Be accepting of challenges and disruptions. Be flexible in your implementation schedule. Maintain your inspiration by working with others, reading, reflecting, and reminding yourself of your motivation statement.

INDEX

ABOUT ONTOS HEALTH RETREAT

Ontos is a 700-acre (280-hectare) idyllic haven for peace and relaxation located in the foothills of the Snowy Mountains outside of Buchan in East Gippsland, Victoria, Australia. One of the few health retreats in the world that provides both family and adults-only times, Ontos offers a complete array of daily programs and services for recharging and rejuvenating the body, mind, and spirit. The health-enhancement focus at Ontos includes stretching, meditation, stress management, and relaxation classes, massage, hiking, Integral Yoga sessions, health talks and workshops, children's stretching/yoga/creativity programs, and more! The Ontos program leaves guests feeling renewed without reliance on fitness machines or fad diets, but rather through an integrated program of health-enhancement activities.

Ontos is also an organic farm that produces much of its own food through extensive orchards, vegetable gardens, hothouses, and broad-scale agriculture. The meals served at Ontos are one of the added attractions, using fresh produce and innovative recipes that are both tasty and healthy. Established in 1980, Ontos has grown with the addition of motel units, a conference center, and an all-faiths temple. It is a unique experience in healthy living, where you can go at your own pace, yet feel the benefits immediately.

Ontos Health Retreat
Buchan Post Office
Victoria Australia 3885

Telephone 61-51-55-0275

THE HELP FOUNDATION, INC.

The HELP Foundation, Inc. was established as a non-profit charitable organization in 1992. It is the goal of the foundation to assist and educate the public on healthy lifestyle issues. The foundation hopes to work through schools and community health centers, with a focus on:

- Imparting a sound understanding of the relevance of nutrition, exercise, communication, meditation, stretching, positive thinking, sharing, creativity, planning, lifestyle, and relaxation to health and well-being

- Disseminating information on disease-prevention measures to the general public

- Providing training for members of the general public and health practitioners to enable them to assist in the delivery of this service to those suffering from debilitating illnesses

- Self-help techniques to assist in the recovery and coping process

The HELP Foundation, Inc. values a close partnership with medical and health professionals. The Health Enhancement Lifestyle Program Ltd is at present the sole source of funding for the HELP Foundation, but it is hoped that further ties with funding groups can be developed.

If you are interested in learning more about the HELP Foundation, contact Neal Hoptman on 61-51-55-0295, or write to the HELP Foundation, c/o Neal Hoptman, Gelantipy Rd, Buchan PO, Victoria 3885, Australia.

THE HEALTH ENHANCEMENT LIFESTYLE PROGRAM

If you have enjoyed HELP Yourself To Health, there are a number of services that you might be interested in:

- HELP Residential Programs—Six-day in-depth lifestyle training programs offered at Ontos Health Retreat frequently throughout the year.

- HELP Outpatient Programs—Ongoing programs available through hospitals that have adopted the Health Enhancement Lifestyle Program.

- HELP for Health Professionals—Training courses for health professionals interested in helping their own patients through a lifestyle program.

- HELP for Business—Short- and long-term in-house or residential training to meet corporate needs.

- HELP Education—Speakers available to make presentations in schools, businesses, community centers, service clubs, and social groups to talk about all aspects of the program and give people an experience of how to help themselves to health.

- HELPful Hints—A newsletter to keep you informed of upcoming HELP events as well as tips to maintain a healthy lifestyle.

- HELP *International*—Training in all aspects of the Health Enhancement Lifestyle Program is now available in the USA. Please contact Neal Hoptman (address and telephone number below) to obtain the latest information about this growing area.

While the residential programs are just one way to access HELP, their effectiveness cannot be overstated. It is highly recommended that all individuals participate in this program if possible.

For further information on any of the services listed, please contact Neal Hoptman on 61-51-55-0295, or write to Neal Hoptman, Health Enhancement Lifestyle Program Ltd, Buchan PO, Victoria 3885, Australia.

HEALTH ENHANCEMENT LIFESTYLE PROGRAM
AUDIOTAPE SERIES

These audiotapes will guide you through the steps necessary to develop greater health through an easeful body, a peaceful mind, and a useful life.

- *Health through Relaxation*—A variety of practical approaches for releasing stress that everyone can immediately benefit from is followed by a guided deep relaxation session. This 60-minute recording is available on CD as well as audiotape.

- *Rejuvenate through Yoga*—This presents an Integral Yoga approach to classic yoga postures and breathing practices to rejuvenate body and mind. A 60-minute comprehensive yoga class guides you through the postures illustrated in *HELP Yourself to Health*.

- *Health through Meditation*—Effective concentration techniques to calm and focus the mind are presented in an easy-to-follow format. Helpful hints for dealing with distraction and challenges in developing your meditation practice are followed by a guided meditation session that you can use daily.

- *Stretch for Health*—This energizing daily routine of stretching, yoga, and relaxation will promote an easeful body. The 45-minute routine is a wonderful way to start your day by limbering up gently with guidance.

These tapes are available individually or together as a complete set. The cost is only AUS$19.95 or US$9.95 each, plus postage. *Health through Relaxation* CD is AUS $24.95 or US $14.95.

To order your tapes or CDs, just phone HELP on 61-51-55-0295, write to HELP Yourself to Health, Ontos Health Retreat, Buchan PO, Buchan, Victoria 3885, Australia, or, for *Health through Relaxation* only, contact:

Millennium Books
E J Dwyer (Australia) Pty Ltd
Locked Bag 71
Alexandria NSW 2015 Australia

Telephone 61-2-550-2355
Facsimile 61-2-519-3218

Notes

Notes

Notes

Notes

Notes

Notes

Notes